Vitamin D: Benefits vs. False Claims

A SELECTIVE REVIEW

Prof Randolph M. Howes MD,PhD

Orthomolecular Scientist, Surgeon, Scholar, Author and Biochemist

Adjunct Assistant Professor of Plastic Surgery, (RET.)
The Johns Hopkins Hospital, Baltimore, MD. USA

Espaldon Professor of Plastic and Reconstructive Surgery,
University of Santo Tomas, Manila, Philippines

Adjunct Professor of Biological Sciences,
Southeastern Louisiana University

Professor of Surgery, Biophysics and Biochemistry,
Louisiana University of Medical Sciences (RET.)

Dean, Louisiana University of Medical Sciences (RET.)

(Also holds an Honorary Doctorate of Humanities)

It is understood that medicine is an ever-changing science. As new research and clinical experience broaden our knowledge, changes in treatment and drug therapy are required. The author and the publisher of this work have checked with sources believed to be reliable in their efforts to provide information that is complete and generally in accord with the standards accepted at the time of publication. However, in view of the possibility of human error or changes in the medical sciences, neither the authors nor the publisher nor any other party who has been involved in the preparation of publication of this work warrants that the information contained herein is in every respect accurate or complete, and they disclaim all responsibility to any errors or omissions or for the results obtained from use of the information contained in the work. Readers should confirm the information contained herein with other sources. For example and in particular, readers are advised to check the product information sheets (or labels) included in the package of each drug they plan to administer to be certain that the information contained in this work is accurate and that changes have not been made in the recommended dose or in the contraindications for administration. This recommendation is of particular importance in connection with new or infrequently used drugs, additives or supplements.

Disclaimers: Please note: only your personal physician or other health professional you consult can best advise you on matters of your health based on your medical history, your family medical history, your medication history, and how information from any of these databases may apply to you. Neither Dr. Howes nor any party involved in creating, producing or delivering this web site shall be liable for any damages arising out of access to or use of this material or web site, or any errors or omissions in the content thereof.

The information given herein is not intended as medical advice. Always consult with your doctor for underlying illness. Before beginning dietary investigation, consult a dietician or a physician with an interest in nutrition. Information is drawn from the scientific literature, web research, and personal enquiry; while all care is taken, information is not warranted as accurate and the author cannot be held liable for any errors and omissions.

Financial disclosure: Dr. Howes has no financial conflicts of interest and is not involved in the sale of dietary supplements or fitness equipment. The author holds no stocks or interests in companies in the food additive or antioxidant supplement business.

My credo:

"I am the one who wishes to be studious,
when others do not want to study,
to be diligent, when others do not want to work
and the one who remains curious for discovery,
whilst others remain pacified.
I am the doer.
I can. I will. I must."
R. M. Howes, M.D., Ph.D.
5/25/04

ABOUT THE AUTHOR
Prof. Randolph M. Howes M.D., Ph.D.

Biographical sketch:

As a champion of the people, Dr. Howes anticipates and hopes for the active involvement of all connected parties (patients, caregivers, healthcare professionals, etc.) as an integral approach to educating consumers and the public about the potential dangers of excessive antioxidant-containing supplements and "antioxidant stacking."

Some people are born with a silver spoon in their mouth but Dr. Howes had to earn his. Even as a child, Dr. Howes could think with adult clarity. He could envision his future but it would require "decades of dedication" to make it a reality.

From childhood, Dr. Howes was motivated to become a medical doctor and scientist. Assuredly, having been born on a small strawberry farm in rural Louisiana, his journey to the top has proved to be arduous and demanding.

However, he was fortunate to acquire the confidence of Sister Elizabeth at St. Joseph's school and went on to gain the support of his high school speech teacher, Mrs. Iris Brann, who also had strong beliefs in his abilities and potential. Ultimately, with the help of his guitar and his singing ability, he defeated the star quarter back of the high school football team to become the president of the student body.

With the aid of a $25 dollar legislative scholarship, he went on to Southeastern Louisiana College (SLC). At SLC, he was selected for honors chemistry, made the Dean's list, worked at the Psychology Research

Lab forty hours a week, maintained a premed study load, and was elected president of the Junior Class and the Interfraternity Council.

To earn badly needed funds, he played music on weekends in a small combo, The Three Blind Mice. Next, he matriculated to Tulane University School of Medicine.

His initial dream was to try to combine both medicine and science. In that regard, he began work as a technician with Dr. Andrew Schally at the Endocrine Polypeptide Lab in the isolation of thyrotropin releasing factor. That work led to a Nobel Prize for Dr. Schally.

Dr. Howes had been highly impressed with the enthusiasm of biochemist, the late Dr. Richard H. Steele, who accepted him as a doctoral candidate under his tutelage. Dr. Howes graduated in the top 10 of his class, won the Louisiana Pathology Association Award, was elected to the Sigma Xi honor fraternity and was the first in the history of Tulane to become a Doctor of Medicine and a Ph.D. in biochemistry concurrently.

Next, he was selected to pursue a career in surgery at the prestigious Johns Hopkins Hospital.

Unbelievably, at Dr. Howes' urging, he was allowed to operate his own research lab during his surgical internship and residency training while at Johns Hopkins Hospital. He worked hand in hand with the greats in American medicine and surgery.

Independently, he garnered grants, trained lab techs, wrote papers, slept on the cold floor, proudly served as a Captain in the U.S. Army Reserves Medical Corp and finished with board eligibility in both general and plastic surgery in an unheard of six year period.

In another first, he was appointed as an Adjunct Assistant Professor of Plastic Surgery at Johns Hopkins Hospital. He retired from that position in 2013.

For decades, Dr. Howes gave unselfishly to pro bono medical missions in the Philippines and he holds the Ernesto Espaldon Chair as Professor of Plastic Surgery at the University of Santo Tomas.

Upon retirement from a career in cosmetic plastic surgery, he is living his dream of trying to revolutionize the treatment of cancer, heart disease, HIV/AIDS and malaria, with his in depth knowledge of the arcane biochemistry of oxygen metabolism. He is a work in progress! Dedicated and passionate, he is on a mission for mankind.

Dr. Howes invented the triple lumen venous catheter, which has been credited with helping save the lives of over 20 million critically ill patients worldwide. His catheter became the number one venous catheter in the world and his name is well recognized in over 100 countries. He has been recognized as a humanitarian, visionary, entrepreneur, singer, songwriter, inventor and author.

He received the Harper Award for innovative research from the American College for Advancement in Medicine, served as their keynote speaker and his peers refer to him as "a walking encyclopedia on oxygen metabolism."

He is a Dr. Norman Vincent Peale Unsung Hero award winner, which recognized his awesome versatility. Additionally, even though he is humble and does not like talking about it, he is a self made multi-millionaire.

He is currently doing extensive research on cures for cancer and heart disease and development of revolutionary treatment modalities. He has written 20 books over the past 8 years on the subject of antioxidants and oxygen metabolism, as it relates to protection from cancer, heart disease, diabetes, malaria, HIV/AIDS, Alzheimer's disease, aging and arthritis. He has written many scientific and medical papers and has lectured nationally and internationally.

His research has shown that currently common antioxidant vitamins, such as vitamins A & E, (and vitamin C to a lesser extent) can be harmful and that oxygen free radicals protect us from bacterial, fungal and viral infections and they help to control cancer growth and metastasis.

He has developed an effective, inexpensive singlet oxygen generating system, from orthomolecular agents, for the treatment of cancer and heart disease. He is passionate about his research and hopes to have his discoveries at the patient's bedside in his lifetime. Admittedly, this is an extremely ambitious goal.

There are over 8,000 pages in his magnum opus and at the Howes World Selective Library on Oxygen Metabolism. Over 3,000 pages of his opus are available online in a searchable format www.iwillfindthe-cure.org © by R.M. Howes

NOTE: An avid researcher, Dr. Howes has authored more than 350 original publications, including over 30 medical and scientific books, such as Death In Small Doses (Antioxidant vitamins A, C & E in the 21st Century), Antioxidant Overkill and Dangers of Excessive Antioxidants In Cancer Patients. He has written numerous articles for medical and consumer publications, including The Journal of American Academy of Cosmetic Surgery, Annals of the New York Academy of Science, The Journal of Evidence Based Complementary And Alternative Medicine, The Baton Rouge Advocate, and The Houma Courier. He has a weekly science/medicine column in the Hammond Daily Star, the Independence Times and The Ponchatoula Times. His research interests include truthful reporting of antioxidant dangers, adverse effects of vitamins A, C & E, other antioxidant's deadly unintended consequences, free radicals, oxygen metabolism, and cancer and heart disease treatment and prevention, global health care policy, and oxidative means to revolutionize treating and preventing HIV/AIDS and malaria.

Dr. Howes is also an active and well-known speaker and media personality, having been featured on PBS's The American Health Journal, WWL-TV New Orleans and WDSU-TV New Orleans, Sirius/XM satellite radio, as well as many other national talk and news shows across America.

In 2013, he received from the American College for Advancement In Medicine the first Charles Farr Award for "excellence in oxidative medicine."
After reading Dr. Howes' book, *Dangers of Excessive Antioxidants In Cancer Patients,* Robert C. Allen, M.D., Ph.D., Chairman of the Department of Pathology at Creighton Medical School in Omaha, Nebraska, described Dr. Howes this way,
"During my forty-five-year association with Dr. Randolph M. Howes, I've been consistently impressed, and sometimes exhausted, by his brilliance, energy and intensity. Over the past several years his attention has been focused on debunking the meme that oxidants are "bad" and antioxidants are "good". We should all appreciate that oxidation provides the energy that drives all complex life forms. *Dangers of Excessive Antioxidants in Cancer Patients* presents convincing arguments with supporting evidence that simplistically assuming antioxidants are somehow "good" is not valid. Dr. Howes is *The Scientific Voyager* poetically described herein, and this book is the product of his voyage."

Dr. Allen answered the question, "If you or a loved one had cancer, would you now take or recommend antioxidants?" He answered, "If I had cancer and was undergoing chemotherapy, I certainly would not be taking BHT, vitamins A and E, or any "antioxidant" formulation, nor would I recommend antioxidants to my family, loved ones, or anyone else." His support of Dr. Howes' work is clear and undeniable.

Following the same scenario, Dr. Robert Muller, M.D. (Ob-Gyn) answered this way: "Dr Howes book shows the extensive research done on antioxidants, BUT the difficulty lies in overcoming the social norms established by the brainwashing of the public by the pharmaceutical industry. If common sense prevails, the choice becomes very clear—antioxidants are worthless in the prevention and treatment of cancer (and CVD)." Robert Muller, M.D. 5-12-11

These are just two examples of highly qualified, medically-involved, individuals who recognize the innovative brilliance of Dr. Howes' new approach to disease prevention, causation and coexistence.

Dr. Howes' origin from a small Louisiana farming community imbedded in him a unique level of morality, ethical behavior and common sense. He feels that common sense is "commonly missing" in the world of medical science today. True, one must be trained to deal with the arcane biological and physiological sciences but one must also be open-minded and willing to rely on common sense, especially when certain scientific theories go against or fly in the face of inductive/deductive reasoning and clear thinking.

Dr. Howes spent over a quarter of a century in educational training to prepare himself for the challenging world of medical science. He is fulfilling his dreams of making significant contributions to the prevention and cure of some of mankind's most deadly diseases, such as cancer, heart disease, malaria and HIV/AIDS.

He feels strongly that he must place his innovative ideas onto the public forum, utilizing printed media and the world wide web. Thus, others can evaluate the validity of his contributions and continue in the pursuit of his dreams.

DEDICATION

To Robin, Don, Sally, Michael, Damien,
Aubrey, Shelby, Cody, Aaron and Michelle,
Clarence, Wendy, John, Shannon, Keith and Noel.

The scientific method demands that we change our beliefs or theories to fit the factual data. I believe that this applies directly to the Free Radi-Crap theory. Again, I say to you, "The free radical theory has fallen and so has the mitochondrial free radical theory of aging."

The unanswerable mysteries
of being alive
are surpassed only by
the incomprehensible mysteries
of being dead.
R. M. Howes, M.D., Ph.D.
10/30/11

Oxygen almost single handedly
fulfilled the possibility of life
on planet Earth.
The proof is all around us.
R. M. Howes, M.D., Ph.D.
8/25/11

THE SCIENTIFIC VOYAGER

The vast immensity of the data ocean surrounds and engulfs
you.
At first, you glimpse something foggy on the far away re-
search horizon.
You diligently pursue, in that direction, to get a better look.
A distant shape is then suggested, but needs considerable
clarification.
You move in, study it intensely - all possibilities, intensively.
An image of enlightenment begins to form.
It has a pattern and design....but is it real or just another
illusion?
More study, more study, more study and
now it congeals into focus. Your mind's eye can see it ever so
clearly.
It is a magnificent island of discovery
jutting out of a raging sea of unknowns.
Now, you must step out onto its slippery rock surface
to be scientifically satiated.
There....you feel it solidly under your feet. Eureka!
But how do you inform others of your discovery?
How do you bring them onshore with you?
Carefully, very, very carefully
for many are still blind,
still uninformed, still misinformed, still lost at sea!
Yet, for you, the tumultuous journey is at an end.
You are scientifically satisfied....
'till you launch the next inquiry.

R. M. Howes, M.D., Ph.D.
4/1/11

Millions have taken antioxidant vitamin supplements religious-
ly for decades truly believing that they were overall healthy
in reducing cancer, heart disease and strokes and extending
their life span, when current evidence clearly shows they are
at best, nearly useless, and at worst, harmful.
(Howes, 2012)

VITAMIN D:
BENEFITS VS. FALSE CLAIMS
TABLE OF CONTENTS:

The U.T.O.P.I.A. Institute and Free Radical Publishing Co.
(Note: The vitamin D referred to throughout this text is D3, unless specified otherwise)

SECTION ONE

INTRODUCTION

Patient Confusion and Medical Conflicts Grow

As regards vitamin D levels and vitamin D deficiency or insufficiency, the optimal serum concentration of vitamin D has not been established and it may change across different stages of life. Similarly, there is currently no consensus on target serum vitamin D levels.

There does, however, appear to be a consensus on the definition of vitamin D deficiency at 25(OH)D < 25 nmol/l, which is based on the risk of diseases such as rickets and osteomalacia. Higher target serum levels have also been proposed based on subclinical endpoints such as parathyroid hormone (PTH). (Health Quality Ontario, 2010)

In Australia, as of 2013, the marked variation in the frequency of **testing for vitamin D deficiency indicates that large sums of potentially unnecessary funds are being expended.** The rate of 25(OH)D testing increased exponentially at an unsustainable rate. Consequences of such findings are widespread in terms of cost and effectiveness. Further research is required to determine the drivers and cost benefit of effectiveness of 25(OH) vitamin D testing. (Bilinski, Boyages, 2013)

Also, please let me interject at the offset, that I feel that the salutary effects of vitamin D, especially as regards cancer and cardiovascular disease are due to its prooxidant activity. I will not get into an extended discussion of this subject in this book but I do refer you to my companion books for in depth discussions of the subject of redox and oxidative medicine.

Here are ten titles to current books on the subject of vitamin D, which champion its alleged miraculous salutary effects on human health. At best, these books are misleading and at worst, they are calculated falsehoods, designed to get money from your pocket into their pocket.

The titles of these books are tailored to put vitamin D in glowing terms, but much of the "shine" has come off of the sunshine vitamin.

A glance at these titles, with their included quips, would make one believe that vitamin D can prevent or cure a wide spectrum of disease pathophysiologies. But, they are wrong. Vitamin D has limited preventative and curative effects according to the best scientific evidence available today.

Just look at this hype!

The Miraculous Results Of Extremely High Doses Of The Sunshine Hormone Vitamin D3 My Experiment With Huge Doses... by Jeff T Bowles - High dose Vitamin D3 therapy over the last year *CURED ALL MY CHRONIC CONDITIONS* - SOME THAT I'D HAD FOR 20+ YEARS!

The Vitamin D Solution: A 3-Step Strategy to Cure Our Most Common Health Problems by Michael F. Holick and Andrew Weil - The vitamin D solution sets a new standard in health and well-ness that I believe will *change the face of medicine* as we know it. Andrew Weil.

The Vitamin D Cure, Revised by James Dowd - We now know that adding vitamin D to your daily regimen can net you *unbelievable benefits*, from reducing your chances of having certain kinds of cancer to gaining flexibility and youthful exuberance well into your seventies and beyond.

VITAMIN D: Miracle Vitamin: The Ultimate Vitamin D Benefit and Cure Guide to Beat Depression, Lose Weight, and... by James Banner - Vitamin D has been called the *"Miracle Vitamin"* due to it's *hundreds of life regenerating properties*.

The Vitamin D Revolution: How the Power of This Amazing Vitamin Can Change Your Life by Soram Khalsa - Recent, groundbreaking medical research has made a connection between Vitamin D deficiency and 17 types of cancers, including breast, colon, and prostate. Illnesses such as influenza, diabetes, multiple sclerosis, and coronary heart disease have also been connected to a lack of this vitamin.

The Vitamin D Miracle: How to Cure Common Health Problems and Have Optimal Health by Vincent Miles - You're about to discover how to have optimal health and_cure numerous common health issues_ simply by getting more of a simple vitamin in your life.

Vitamin D Explained: The Incredible, Healing Powers of Sunlight by C.K. Murray - High blood pressure, heart disease, diabetes, allergies, depression, and even cancer can _all be treated_ through Vitamin D.

Vitamin D: Is This the Miracle Vitamin? by Ian Wishart - Vitamin D is _the hottest development in medical science._

The Secrets of Vitamin D in Weight Loss and Disease Prevention by Mir Joffrey - Vitamin D has been associated with _potentially preventing disease ranging from the flu to cancer_ due to its role in the immune system.

Prescribing Sunshine: Why vitamin D should be flying off shelves by M. Aziz - Vitamin D is shaping up to become _the greatest natural health intervention of all time_.

After reviewing the current scientific literature concerning vitamin D, I can say that it is definitely not miraculous, even though it does have some redeeming properties.

Also, the terms "prevent" and "cure" are thrown around with reckless abandon. This is in violation of the DSHEA Act of 1994, which makes it illegal for supplement marketers and profiteers to use the terms "treat," "diagnose," "prevent," or "cure."

Query: But, who is going to stop them?

Answer: No one.

For years, I have written of how patients are bombarded with confusing medical articles and that we have arrived at a point where common sense has collided with so-called medical science.

As a patient advocate, I carefully follow the medical literature addressing the harmful potential of pharmaceutical drugs and supplements. There are so many drug related complications coming out on a daily basis, that it is difficult to keep up and full disclosure by the drug companies is still a far away goal and manipulation of their drug data, to increase sales, is commonplace.

The unacceptable annual number of deaths (over 106,000 annually) from drug adverse effects must be addressed. We are in an age in which snake oil flows faster than Texas crude.

The entire dietary supplement industry is out of control, with over 55,000 being peddled, and our citizens are paying premium prices for in-effective and potentially harmful chemical concoctions tagged as "medi-cal breakthroughs" and "magic pills."

We are witnessing conflicting and opposing recommendations on breast mammography, cervical PAP smears, desired blood pressure levels, safe levels of cholesterol, blood pressure cut off points for hypertension, safety of saturated and polyunsaturated fats, etc. And a major debate can not decide on what really constitutes a so-called "healthy diet."

Still, there are now governmental mandates, directing the "food police" on what you can eat, even though the long-standing food pyramid was recently scrapped and replaced by the new and improved food "pie chart."

And don't even go to the area of weight loss. Even Dr. Oz's daily hour-long infomercial can't make consistent recommendations and guide-lines, without pushing tons of questionable supplements on uninformed viewers. This only leads to patient confusion and skepticism regarding any and all medical recommendations.

Just look at the panic of our population created by false alarms (national emergencies) regarding the yearly flu epidemics, or the ineffectiveness of our vaccination programs. An even larger looming problem is the fact that medical intervention can "sustain" life, even when quality is totally gone, for indefinite or extended costly periods.

As government controlled healthcare takes over, so called "death pan-els" may be as close as the Veterans Administration Hospitals. And, so-cialized medicine is as close as the Affordable Care Act (Obamacare), which will bring a new low of patient care quality to all of our citizenry (President and Congress exempted, of course).

Without meaningful tort reform, healthcare costs will continue to spi-ral out of control and where will all of the "new doctors" come from to take care of an additional thirty million people?

In the America that I love, I continually shake my head at the bleak medical picture presented by the daily news. Folks, brace yourself for the medical "new normal."

Vitamin D deficiency

It seems that when many of today's physicians are left without a diagnosis, they assign the diagnosis of "vitamin D deficiency" on this large group of patients and their underlying, unknown illnesses.

Television ads promote testosterone supplements for "low T" and others push vitamin D.

Nearly 30% of the world population is overweight or obese. **The obesity epidemic is global: 2.1 billion people, or about 29% of the world's population in 2013.**

The incidence of overweight and obesity rose by 27.5% for adults and 47.1% for children between 1980 and 2013, according to researchers at the Institute for Health Metrics and Evaluation at the University of Washington and published in the *Lancet*.

Cancer and heart disease are on the rise and a multitude of other diseases continues to increase. Could some of these conditions be caused by **a vitamin D deficiency**? More and more, American physicians are labeling patients with a diagnosis of vitamin D deficiency.

But just how much of this medical dogma is true?

Recent controversy over figures used in the British Medical Journal which were later withdrawn renewed **questions over the peer review system** - the way medical studies are checked prior to publication.

The system used to check papers before they appear in journals is called peer review.

It is a way of validating their work through the scrutiny of the methodology that was used by other experts.

There is an increasing problem in the scientific community: a dramatic increase in the number of papers retracted or taken back by journals. When a paper is retracted, it means that the research has so many flaws that it has to be withdrawn by the publications in question. Many consider this action as the worst punishment for a scientist.

The number of retractions has increased dramatically - in 2000 there were 30 but in 2010 this number had risen to 400. But, **these**

retractions still represent 0.35% of what is published each year - around 1.4 million studies.

Retraction of papers recently happened concerning articles published about the effectiveness of the antioxidant, resveratrol, for increasing longevity. Much of the data was falsified.

When there has been an "inappropriate handling of data," the work should be retracted. **Peer reviews aren't exempt from problems. However, the literature often does not correct itself. RMH Note: such is the case with the free radical theory.** (Please refer to my books in the reference section or check them out at www.amazon.com)

This should apply to the free radical theory of so-called anti-oxidants. Repeated studies have shown it to be invalid, thus, the original papers should be pulled from print or duly noted that they have been debunked.

There is evidence that researchers sometimes selectively present data that supports a specific hypothesis and I have never seen such biased studies as those involving free radicals and antioxidant dietary supplements.

According to a 2009 PLOS article, about 2% of scientists have admitted to falsifying, making up or modifying elements at least once.

And **one third confessed to other "questionable practices", including "to have 'modified research results' to improve the outcome, then to have reported results they 'knew to be untrue'."**

Additionally, **more than 70% of scientists say they have witnessed irregular behavior from their colleagues.**

Further, it has been said that "Wikipedia, the online encyclo-pedia, contains errors in nine out of 10 of its health entries, and should be treated with caution."

The open-access nature has "raised concern" among doctors about its reliability, as **Wikimedia UK is the sixth most popular site on the internet. Reportedly, up to 70% of physicians and medical students use the tool.**

Confusing times, medically speaking

Americans are regularly presented with confusing and conflicting healthcare data. We are cautioned against breathing pollutant-containing air, eating mercury laced fish, consuming harmful processed sugar, ingesting saturated fats in meats, buying trans fat-containing snack foods, gulping down any type of fast (junk) food and drinking water with hidden contaminants of hormones, drug residues, pesticides or herbicides.

Yet, man's average life span continues to increase. This can be a difficult situation to sort out, even for those of us in the medical/scientific field.

Even more worrisome is the nearly unrestrained marketing for pharmaceuticals. Drug advertisements are made more palatable by the inclusion of pretty little carpenter bees, cute butterflies or rainbows, while potentially lethal side effects are hurriedly glossed over.

Effective television and radio drug ads, selected by focus groups, are constantly pushing consumers to prod their physicians to prescribe their newer products.

Sixty Minutes showed a re-run of the deplorable tactics of the pharmaceutical industry in passage of the unbelievably costly 2003 Medicare Modernization (Drug) Act. The complicity, with then Senator Billy Tauzin and many other elected and government officials, who shortly thereafter became handsomely paid employees of the drug industry, was a shameless assault on our taxpayers. In fact, it was an outrage, but just one of many.

Yet, neither our Democrat nor Republican elected officials were capable (or willing) of protecting their constituents. On the floors of congress, money talks loudly, whilst deals are cut with whispered arrangements.

Even though all of us are vulnerable to clever and subliminal advertising techniques, we should seriously consider scientific studies, which point out the dangers in using many current medications and dietary supplements for treating diabetes, depression and heart disease.

Patient's Confusion with Drugs

A procession of pharmaceutical caveats and warnings are issued on a regular basis concerning popular medications. To wit, Nexium is the third biggest selling drug in the world, behind the cholesterol medicine Lipitor and blood thinner Plavix, with global sales totaling $5.7 billion in 2005.

Taking such popular heartburn drugs as Nexium, Prevacid or Prilosec for a year or more can raise the risk of a broken hip markedly in people over 50.

The patients who used these proton pump inhibitors for more than a year had a 44 percent higher risk of hip fracture than nonusers. The longer the patients took the drugs, the higher their risk. The study found a similar risk of hip fractures for drugs called H2 blockers, which includes Tagamet and Pepcid.

Two Parkinson's disease drugs cause the same kind of heart damage that led to the withdrawal of the diet drug combination "fen-phen."

Patients taking the drugs pergolide, (Permax), and cabergoline (Dostinex), had a sharply higher risk of heart valve damage than those taking other therapies. Pergolide is also used to treat restless leg syndrome.

Wyeth Pharmaceuticals recalled their drugs fenfluramine, or Pondimin, and dexfenfluramine, or Redux in 1997 after some of the 6 million Americans who had taken fen-phen developed heart-valve problems.

The current cavalcade of patient confusion, such as that seen with hormone replacement therapy, leads to angst towards all medications.

We must endeavor to inform patients and to strive for utmost patient safety. Thus, I have written extensively on the harmful potential of common dietary supplements, including vitamin D.

Bias and Omissions Plague Medical Research

Common tactics or tricks used by drug and supplement manufacturers (or those selling these products) are to either ignore negative results or to deny their existence.

The Institute for Quality and Efficiency in Health Care (IQWiG) in Germany has reviewed research and found that this applies to all sorts of conditions, including depression, Alzheimer's disease, type 2 diabetes, menopausal symptoms and cancer.

Beate Wieseler, deputy head of IQWiG's Drug Assessment Department, said, "It's widespread, and it affects drug companies, universities and regulatory authorities."

Supplement manufacturers, such as with antioxidant vitamins (including vitamin D), routinely, and legally, sell their products without first having to demonstrate that they are safe and effective. The Food and Drug Administration has not made full use of even the limited authority granted it by the industry-friendly 1994 Dietary Supplement Health and Education Act (DSHEA).

To date, it has required only one ingredient to be taken off the market, i.e., ephedrine alkaloids, and this followed decades of debate.

For 13 years after the enactment of the DSHEA, supplement makers didn't have to tell the FDA of serious side effects but this was finally corrected by a law that closed that loophole and took effect in December 2007.

Because of inadequate quality control and inspection, supplements contaminated with heavy metals, pesticides, or prescription drugs have been sold to unsuspecting consumers (victims).

Further, Food and Drug Administration (FDA) rules covering manufacturing quality do not apply to the companies that supply herbs, vitamins, and other raw ingredients. Many of these vitamins and supplements are made in China and the FDA has failed to inspect even one of these manufacturers as of 2010. Hidden or misleading studies may represent a huge threat to all of us.

Frequently, medical journals or pharmaceutical companies that sponsor research will report only "positive" results, leaving out the non-findings or negative findings where a new drug or procedure may have proved more harmful than helpful.

This problem particularly arises when pharmaceutical, supplement or medical device companies fund so-called medical studies, because there is a "curious association" between industry sponsorship and positive outcomes or conclusions in studies.

We must correct the situation whereby patients may not know the full story about their drugs or their medical treatments because of a widespread problem involving unpublished or biased clinical trials.

We must demand full disclosure on all of these drug and supplement products. Then, and only then, will people be able to decide for themselves if they are going to take these products. Such is the case with vitamin D.

Down with the snake oil salesmen and up with truth.

Can We Trust Medical Studies Today?

Medical news reports and articles are to be approached with an eye of skepticism. We have found that so-called scientific studies can be seriously "doctored" to produce an advantageous result, which is usually directed by a profit motive.

As the old maxim goes, "Follow the money."

Dr. Catherine DeAngelis, editor of the Journal of the American Medical Association (JAMA), recently said, "Misleading research is often published in major medical journals and doctors are lending their names to it.

Doctors, regulators, publishers and others are all taking money, information and small presents from pharmaceutical companies and being influenced in the process."

Dr. John Santa, a medical consultant to Consumers Union, said "Pharmaceutical companies need to get out of the business of 'ghostwriting' articles for medical journals."

JAMA presented Merck's Vioxx case as a specific example of the problem, in which data showing that Vioxx harmed patients was suppressed and academic researchers had lent credibility to the company's allegedly manipulated research by putting their names on the work.

In short, DeAngelis said there is a "gigantic" problem of drug companies influencing doctors and patients. Drug companies conduct "campaigns of persuasion" and spend millions upon millions of dollars on promotional materials, pens, prescription pads, honoraria, consulting fees, travel expenses and booths at major medical meetings. They pay physicians to travel to seminars, often in exotic places, to learn about their latest drug push. They send articulate and attractive drug representatives and "detailers" to pay personal visits to doctors.

The situation is even worse when it comes to dietary supplements, including vitamin D.

Also, the drug companies fund many medical studies. DeAngelis said, "We have given away our profession and we have got to take it back. The influence does not usually amount to outright bribery. We just have to be more careful, all of us, and insist that we are not going to be hoodwinked by them, fooled by them."

We must remember that physicians took a sworn oath to their patients and not to the drug companies. Doctors must constantly re-earn the respect and trust given to them by the good deeds of previous honorable physicians.

Doctors must not let their medical judgment be clouded by financial interests and must be guided by the patient's needs and their safety. That is the bottom line. Sadly, many doctors, including ole' Dr. Oz, are seemingly led by the profit motive, when it comes to their endorsement of various dietary supplements.

Recent research suggests that simply eating an apple a day might help prevent cardiovascular -related deaths in those over 50 to a similar degreee as using a daily statin. Even if a drug is backed by scientific evidence, it in no way guarantess its safety or effectiveness.

Similarly, if an alternative treatment has not been published in peer-reviewed medical journal, it does not mean it is unsafe or ineffective. Such seems to be the case with vitamin D.

But, not all the news is grim. Some dietary supplements actually might be of value. Of the 55,000 new supplements on the market, three might be of benefit for otherwise healthy people: calcium and vitamin D in postmenopausal women, to prevent bone thinning; and folic acid during pregnancy, to prevent birth defects.

Background

Over the past six years, I have written medical editorials on the status of vitamin D and they show a progression in our feelings about facts and false claims. Let's start with those for a chronological general overview as to how the vitamin D story has evolved.

MY LETTERS TO EDITOR

Letter to the editor: The Pundit Speaks 2-23-08

Vitamin D3: The Good News 2-23-08

Vitamin D3 (cholecalciferol), which helps with calcium absorption, is consistently reported as being of great benefit to overall good health and has been fortified in milk since 1933 to prevent rickets.

Estimates are that one in 4 people over age 60 have low vitamin D levels, but estimates do vary, depending upon the source.

Sunlight triggers the synthesis of vitamin D in the skin, and people who get little sun exposure tend to have lower stores of the vitamin.

Some studies have shown that rates of breast, colon, ovarian, prostate, pancreatic and lymphomatous cancers are lower in patients with higher vitamin D levels and vitamin D helps prevent cancer cells from growing and spreading.

Other clinical trials in which people were given high doses of vitamin D showed lower risks of cancer, arthritis and diabetes. I believe that this is due to its pro-oxidant activity.

Researchers believe (actually guess) that 60,000 cases of colon cancer and 85,000 cases of breast cancer could be prevented every year in the U.S. for those who maintain a vitamin D level of at least 55 ng/mL. This could be best achieved with a combination of diet, supplements and short intervals of 10 to 15 minutes a day in the sun.

However, we are cautioned to limit sun light exposure because it can lead to skin cancer. Vitamin D is essential for the maintenance of calcium homeostasis and is indicated in combination with calcium to prevent and treat osteoporosis.

Vitamin D also improves muscle strength and function in older adults.

University of California San Diego investigators recommend that, in addition to modest sun exposure, adults get up to 2,000 IU of vitamin D per day, which is the "tolerable upper intake level" set by U.S. health officials.

As with everything, too much can be a bad thing and can increase the risk of vitamin D toxicity, which can cause elevated calcium levels, nausea, weight loss, fatigue and kidney dysfunction.

As a patient advocate, I will recommend safe, readily available and affordable means to improving and maintaining our health and that of our loved ones. Presently, maintaining an adequate intake of vitamin D3 may be one such approach, but the data is shaky on its overall benefits. Letter to the editor: The Pundit Speaks 5-21-09

Vitamin D: Is it a Superstar? 5-21-09

Study after study has supported the importance of maintaining adequate levels of vitamin D3. Repeatedly, reliable studies have linked vitamin D deficiency (low levels) with an increased risk of hypertension, obesity, diabetes, heart attack, stroke and some types of cancer.

On the other hand, patients with adequate vitamin D3 levels have lower rates of breast, colon, ovarian, prostate, pancreatic and lymphomatous cancers.

If that isn't enough, higher vitamin D levels appear to help prevent cancer cells from growing and spreading.

Unbelievably, other studies have shown that people who were given high doses of vitamin D showed lower risks of arthritis and diabetes.

Studies at the University of Manchester have just shown that men, who had higher levels of vitamin D, performed better on memory and information processing tests. In other words, those with higher vitamin D levels were better thinkers.

The team therefore linked vitamin D to higher cognitive performance. Even after calculating for health and lifestyle factors, vitamin D still appeared to be a "brain-power booster." The mechanism of this boost is unknown but I believe that it is due to the strong prooxidant activity of vitamin D3, even though some theorize that its beneficial effects are due to increased antioxidant activity.

Years of intense study lead me to discount the antioxidant theory, especially when one takes into account the essential need for oxygen in normal brain function. In fact, the brain is a sponge for oxygen, since it weighs only 2% of the body's weight but it uses 20% of the oxygen we inhale.

Adequate vitamin D levels are best achieved with a combination of diet (consumption of oily fish), supplements and short intervals of 10 to 15 minutes a day in the sun. However, please remember that there is no such thing as a "healthy sun burn."

Avoid over exposure to the sun and take up to 2,000 IU of vitamin D per day, which is the "tolerable upper intake level" set by U.S. health officials. I have a high level of skepticism on all so-called wonder drugs but vitamin D is seemingly approaching superstar status.

In the America that I love, we will take great interest in medical products which have low toxicity, low risk/benefit ratios and high probabilities of maintaining good health while preventing disease. At present, vitamin D appears to be a "rising star" but only time will tell and if vitamin D studies take a nose dive, you can trust that I will be the first to tell you.

Letter to the editor: The Pundit Speaks 7-1-11

Vitamin D To The Rescue...Again 7-1-11

In December 2010, we were told by the Institute of Medicine, "There's no proof that megadoses of vitamin D prevent cancer or other ailments."

The Institute's two-year study concluded that research into the possible role of vitamin D in other diseases is conflicting, with some studies showing no effect and others showing harm.

However, this flies in the face of the studies from 2007-2009. Prior studies have shown that rates of breast, colon, ovarian, prostate, pancreatic and lymphomatous cancers are lower in patients with higher vitamin D levels and vitamin D helps prevent cancer cells from growing and spreading.

Clinical trials in which people were given high doses of vitamin D showed lower risks of cancer, arthritis and diabetes.

I have attributed this to its prooxidant properties (not antioxidant properties).

Vitamin D3 (cholecalciferol), which helps with calcium absorption, has rather consistently been reported as being of great benefit to overall good health and has been fortified in milk since 1933 to prevent rickets.

Vitamin D improves muscle strength and function in older adults.

Estimates or "guestimates" are that one in 4 people over age 60 have low vitamin D levels.

Sunlight triggers the synthesis of vitamin D (the "sunshine" vitamin) in the skin, and people who get little sun exposure tend to have lower stores of the vitamin. In America, 2,000 IU of vitamin D per day, is the "tolerable upper intake level" set by U.S. health officials.

However, the U.S. Institute of Medicine now recommends 600 IU of vitamin D daily and states as little as 400 IU of vitamin D daily may be protective.

Women most at risk of developing the life-threatening cancer (melanoma) are those who have had a previous non-melanoma form of skin cancer, such as basal cell or squamous cell cancer, and a new study found that the risk for developing melanoma may be cut in half by taking vitamin D/calcium supplements.

The seven year study on 36,282 women was published in the *Journal of Clinical Oncology* and the melanoma risk reduction was not seen among women who had not had an earlier non-melanoma skin cancer. In the United States, more than 68,000 cases of melanoma are diagnosed in adults each year, according to the U.S. National Cancer Institute.

Vitamin D can come from the diet, sun exposure and supplements. Fatty fish and fortified dairy products are two good dietary sources of vitamin D.

In the America that I love, as of 2011, maintaining an adequate intake of prooxidant vitamin D3 appears to be one approach to maintaining good health, that is safe, readily available and affordable.

However, my new book, *Antioxidant Overkill,* (available at Amazon.com) presents overwhelming scientific evidence of the potential harm of antioxidant vitamins A, C and E supplements.

Letter to the editor: The Pundit Speaks 9-4-11

Vitamin D3 Lowers Cancer Risk....Again 9-4-11

Vitamin D3 (cholecalciferol, the form we use in the body), which helps with calcium absorption, has been reported as being of overall benefit to good health.

Sunlight activates the synthesis of vitamin D in the skin, and people who get little sun exposure have lower stores of the vitamin. Patients with higher vitamin D levels have been shown to have lower rates of breast, colon, ovarian, prostate, pancreatic and lymphomatous cancers and vitamin D helps prevent cancer cells from growing and spreading.

Overall, clinical trials in which people were given high doses of vitamin D showed lower risks of cancer, arthritis and diabetes. Interestingly, experts are still at a loss to explain the mechanism of these differences but they have not considered D3's prooxidant character. I have attributed its anti-cancer properties to its prooxidant activity.

U.S. health officials set 2,000 IU of vitamin D per day as the "tolerable upper intake level" but the Institute of Medicine recommends as little as 400 IU daily and concluded there isn't enough information to justify increasing recommended intakes of vitamin D.

Yet, the August 2011 issue of the Journal of Clinical Oncology reported that both higher vitamin D intake and higher blood levels of the vitamin's active form are linked to lower risk of colon and rectal cancers. In 18 studies, on more than 10,000 people, colon cancer risk was as much as 33% lower in subjects with the highest blood levels of vitamin D compared to those with the lowest levels.

Also, when looking at supplements and food as the source of vitamin D, those with the highest intake had 12% lower risk than those with the lowest intakes.

One investigator said, "Up to 58 percent of U.S. adults and adolescents may have vitamin D deficiency, which is "an important health problem in the industrial world."

It is estimated that nearly 37% of Americans take vitamin D supplements.

Arguments rage as to the safest way to get adequate levels of vitamin D. Some say to get it through the diet, while others say to get it by exposure to sunlight, even though sun-exposure is known to increase the risk of skin cancer. Nearly 20% of Americans will develop skin cancer in their lifetime.

In the America that I love, we realize that these findings still need to be confirmed in large, gold-standard randomized clinical trials (RCTs) of vitamin D supplements. Non-melanoma skin cancers are the most common malignant tumor in the U.S. and are diagnosed more than prostate, lung, colorectal, ovarian and breast cancer combined.

As always, use good ole' common sense concerning your health.

Letter to the editor: The Pundit Speaks 7-8-12

Vitamin D3 is Safe and Affordable 7-8-12

For the past four years, I have been telling you of the benefits of vitamin D3. But, please keep in mind the fact that vitamin D3 is more of a pro-hormone than it is a so-called vitamin. In short, it was named incorrectly.

More importantly, it has repeatedly been shown to have low toxicity, low risk/benefit ratios and high probabilities of maintaining good health while preventing disease.

Reliable scientific studies have linked vitamin D deficiency (low levels) with an increased risk of hypertension, obesity, diabetes, heart attack, stroke and some types of cancer. On the other hand, patients with adequate vitamin D3 levels have lower rates of breast, colon, ovarian, prostate, pancreatic and lymphomatous cancers and higher vitamin D levels appear to help prevent cancer cells from growing and spreading.

Still, other studies have shown that people who were given high doses of vitamin D showed lower risks of arthritis and diabetes. Vitamin D3 (cholecalciferol), which helps with calcium absorption, is consistently reported as being of great benefit to overall good health and has been fortified in milk since 1933 to prevent rickets.

Sunlight triggers the synthesis of vitamin D in the skin, and people who get little sun exposure tend to have lower stores of the vitamin. Vitamin D is essential for the maintenance of calcium homeostasis and is indicated in combination with calcium to prevent and treat osteoporosis and fracturing of bones.

Vitamin D also improves muscle strength and function in older adults.

Studies at the University of Manchester have shown that men, who had higher levels of vitamin D, performed better on memory and information processing tests. In other words, those with higher vitamin D levels were better thinkers.

Prof Randolph M. Howes MD,PhD

Adequate levels of vitamin D3 can be maintained by a combination of diet, supplements and short intervals of 10 to 15 minutes a day in the sun. University of California San Diego investigators recommend that, in addition to modest sun exposure, adults get up to 2,000 IU of vitamin D per day, which is the "tolerable upper intake level" set by U.S. health officials.

As with everything, too much can be a bad thing and can increase the risk of vitamin D toxicity but vitamin D3 may still look like a rising star, as of 2012.

I have repeatedly raised cautions against the overuse of the antioxidant vitamins but vitamin D3 may not be in that category. In fact, I believe that it is a good prooxidant. Stay healthy.

Letter to the Editor: The Pundit Speaks 3-13-13

Vitamin D3: The Overall Picture 3-13-13

The term "vitamin" is usually refers to vital substances the body cannot synthesize on its own. Given cholesterol and sunshine, the body can synthesize its own vitamin D. Thus, technically, it is not an essential dietary vitamin.

When it comes to bone health, a meta-analysis showed that high doses of vitamin D lower the risk for fracture by 14% to 30% in people age 65 years or older and one study suggested that low levels of vitamin D increase the risk for forearm fracture in children.

Randomized controlled trials (RCTs) suggested that vitamin D supplementation reduced acute respiratory tract infections in children during the cold Mongolian winter and showed that vitamin D reduced symptoms and antibiotic use in a group of patients with an increased frequency of respiratory infections (colds).

But, a third RCT showed no effect of vitamin D on reducing the incidence or severity of colds in healthy adults.

Low levels of vitamin D have been linked to children with type1 diabetes who have low levels of vitamin D.

Soldiers and women, who have low vitamin D levels during their first trimester of pregnancy, were more likely to develop diabetes.

Epidemiologic studies suggest that a low vitamin D level increases the risk for cardiovascular disease but, an RCT among older women failed to find evidence that vitamin D supplementation improved markers of heart health.

Adequate levels of vitamin D are associated with less weight gain among women age 65 and older.

Vitamin D has been tied to several higher neurological functions and studies have linked autism to low vitamin D during pregnancy, a connection that was strengthened by a map showing that autism rates were highest among children living in states with the lowest levels of sunshine.

People with Alzheimer's disease tend to have low levels of vitamin D, and better cognitive test results are linked to higher vitamin D levels.

Three studies, published in the journal *Neurology*, linked low levels of vitamin D to multiple sclerosis.

Women with sufficient vitamin D levels at baseline are 62% less likely to develop Crohn's disease.

However, for chronic obstructive pulmonary (lung) disease, the story isn't as clear cut.

Vitamin D deficiency is almost universal among patients with chronic kidney disease (CKD) and D3 protects patients undergoing dialysis.

Low vitamin D is linked to food allergy and the list goes on. Of particular interest to me, vitamin D3 is a good prooxidant and not an antioxidant. The "tolerable upper intake level" set by U.S. health officials is up to 2,000 IU of vitamin D per day.

In the America that I love, vitamin D3 seems safe and affordable, as of 2013, for maintaining your health. Yet, there are no unambiguous answers or "magic pills."

Now, let's review general background material on vitamin D.

Vitamin D: An Evidence-Based Review (Kulie et al, 2009)

Although this Kulie et al. review was done in 2009, I have included it in a slightly modified form because it is all inclusive and well referenced.

Vitamin D is a fat-soluble vitamin that plays an important role in bone metabolism and seems to have some anti-inflammatory and immune-modulating properties.

In addition, recent epidemiologic studies have observed relationships between low vitamin D levels and multiple disease states. Low vitamin D levels are associated with increased overall and cardiovascular mortality, cancer incidence and mortality, and autoimmune diseases such as multiple sclerosis.

Although it is well known that the combination of vitamin D and calcium is necessary to maintain bone density as people age, vitamin D may also be an independent risk factor for falls among the elderly.

New recommendations from the American Academy of Pediatrics address the need for supplementation in breastfed newborns and many questions are raised regarding the role of maternal supplementation during lactation. Unfortunately, little evidence guides clinicians on when to screen for vitamin D deficiency or effective treatment options.

Vitamin D is a hormone precursor that is present in 2 forms.

Ergocalciferol, or vitamin D_2, is present in plants and some fish.

Cholecalciferol, or vitamin D_3, is synthesized in the skin by sunlight. Humans can fulfill their vitamin D requirements by either ingesting vitamin D or being exposed to the sun for enough time to produce adequate amounts.

Vitamin D controls calcium absorption in the small intestine and works with parathyroid hormone to mediate skeletal mineralization and maintain calcium homeostasis in the blood stream.

In addition, recent **epidemiologic studies** have observed relationships between low vitamin D levels and multiple disease states, probably caused by its anti-inflammatory and immune-modulating properties and possible affects on cytokine levels.

Vitamin D_3 can be manufactured in the skin by way of ultraviolet (UV) B rays. UVB rays are present only during midday at higher latitudes and do not penetrate clouds. The time needed to produce adequate vitamin D from the skin depends on the strength of the UVB rays (i.e., place of residence), the length of time spent in the sun, and the amount of pigment in the skin.

Tanning beds provide variable levels of UVA and UVB rays and are therefore not a reliable source of vitamin D.

Vitamin D_3 is synthesized from 7-dehydrocholesterol in the skin. The vitamin D binding protein transports the vitamin D_3 to the liver where it undergoes hydroxylation to **25(OH)D (the inactive form of vitamin D) and then to the kidneys where it is hydroxylated by the enzyme 1 αhydroxylase to 1,25(OH)D, its active form**.

This enzyme is also present in a variety of extrarenal sites, including osteoclasts, skin, colon, brain, and macrophages, which may be the cause of it's broad-ranging effects. **The half-life of vitamin D in the liver is approximately 3 weeks**, which underscores the need for frequent replenishment of the body's supply.

Vitamin D and Mortality

Vitamin D may be a determinant of mortality because of its anti-inflammatory and immune-modulating effects. It has been used to treat secondary hyperparathyroidism in people on dialysis. **Retrospective trials show that vitamin D supplementation is associated with decreased mortality in people on dialysis.** (Wolf et al, 2007)

Low serum vitamin D levels are also related to increased mortality in most patients with chronic kidney disease before dialysis. (Inaquma et al, 2008)

However, there have been no randomized prospective trials examining this relationship as of 2007. (Al-Aly, 2007)

In patients not on dialysis, low vitamin D levels are associated with increased levels of inflammation and oxidative load. A prospective study of more than 3,000 male and female patients scheduled for coronary angiography found a positive association between low vitamin D levels and cardiovascular as well as all-cause mortality. (Dobnig et al, 2008)

Data analysis from the National Health and Nutrition Examination Survey III (more than 13,000 adults) showed that people with vitamin D levels in the lowest quartile had a mortality rate ratio of 1.26 (95% CI, 1.08–1.46).

A 2007 meta-analysis demonstrated that intake of a vitamin D supplement at normal doses also was associated with decreased all-cause mortality rates. (Autier, Gandini, 2007)

These data suggest that vitamin D may play a part in multiple causes of death, although causality has not been determined.

Prof Randolph M. Howes MD,PhD

Vitamin D and Cardiovascular Disease

Vitamin D receptors are present in vascular smooth muscle, endothelium, and cardiomyocytes and may have an impact on cardiovascular disease.

Observational studies have shown a relationship between low vitamin D levels and blood pressure, coronary artery calcification, and existing cardiovascular disease. A large cohort study that included more than 1,700 participants from the Framingham offspring study looked at vitamin D levels and incident cardiovascular events. (Wang et al, 2008)

During a period of 5 years, participants who had **25-OH D levels of <15 were more likely to experience cardiovascular events** (hazard ratio, 1.62; 95% CI, 1.11–2.36). The relationship remained significant among people with hypertension but not among those without hypertension. (Wang et al, 2008)

Vitamin D and Diabetes

Recent studies in animal models and humans have suggested that **vitamin D may also play a role in the homeostasis of glucose metabolism and the development of type 1 and type 2 diabetes mellitus (DM).** Epidemiologic data has long suggested a link between exposure to vitamin D early in life and the development of type 1 DM.

Vitamin D_3 receptors have strong immune-modulating effects. In some populations the development of type 1 DM is associated with polymorphisms in the vitamin D receptor gene. There is also some evidence that increased vitamin D intake by infants may reduce the risk of the development of type 1 DM.

Vitamin D has recently been associated with several of the contributing factors known to be linked to the development of type 2 DM, including defects in pancreatic β cell function, insulin sensitivity, and systemic inflammation. Several physiologic mechanisms have been proposed, including the effect of vitamin D on insulin secretion, the direct effect of calcium and vitamin D on insulin action, and the role of this hormone in cytokine regulation.

Although most studies indicating this relationship are observational, **one meta-analysis showed a relatively consistent association between low vitamin D status, calcium or dairy intake, and prevalence of type 2 DM or metabolic syndrome.** The study concluded that the highest type 2 DM prevalence, 0.36, among participants who were not black was associated with the lowest blood levels of 25-hydroxyvitamin D. In addition, metabolic syndrome prevalence of 0.71 was highest among those with the lowest dairy intake. There was also an inverse relationship between type 2 DM and metabolic syndrome incidences and vitamin D and calcium intake. (Pittas et al, 2007)

Vitamin D and Osteoporosis

Osteoporosis is the most common metabolic bone disease in the world. A low vitamin D level is an established risk factor for osteoporosis. **Inadequate serum vitamin D levels will decrease the active transcellular absorption of calcium.**

Although combination calcium and vitamin D supplementation is associated with higher bone mineral density and decreased incidence of hip fractures, the evidence for vitamin D supplementation alone is less clear.

A 2008 evidence summary found that vitamin D supplementation at doses of more than 700 IU daily (plus calcium) prevented bone loss compared with placebo. (Cranney et al, 2008)

However, vitamin D supplementation (300 to 400 IU daily) without calcium did not affect fractures.

A 2005 Cochrane review found unclear evidence that vitamin D alone affected hip, vertebral, or other fracture rates but supported the use of vitamin D with calcium in frail, elderly nursing home residents. (Avenell et al, 2005)

A subsequent 2007 meta-analysis of trials looking at vitamin D and fracture rates concurred that calcium was also necessary to affect a significant difference. (Bonnen et al, 2007)

The recent 2009 meta-analysis of 12 randomized, controlled trials that included more than 42,000 people found that vitamin D supplementation of more than 400 IU daily slightly reduced incidence of nonvertebral fractures (rate ratio, 0.86; 95% CI, 0.77–0.96). (Bischoff-Ferrari et al, 2009)

The effect was dose dependent and was not significant if doses were ≤400 IU daily.

Prof Randolph M. Howes MD, PhD

Vitamin D and Falls among the Elderly

Vitamin D status is increasingly recognized as an important factor in fall status among elderly patients. **Several trials have demonstrated that vitamin D supplementation decreases the risk of falling**. One proposed mechanism is that higher vitamin D levels are associated with improved muscle function.

A 2008 randomized, controlled trial from Australia evaluated women with at least one fall in the preceding 12 months and with a plasma 25-hyroxyvitamin D level <24.0 ng/mL. (Prince et al, 2008)

All women were given calcium 1000 mg per day and were randomized to receive either ergocalciferol 1000 IU per day or placebo. **Women in the study group had fewer falls after 12 months, but this was not a significant difference** (53% versus 62.9%; odds ratio, 0.66; 95% CI, 0.41–1.06). After correction for height difference in the 2 groups, the ergocalciferol group had a significantly lower risk of falling (odds ratio, 0.61; 95% CI, 0.37–0.99).

A dose of 800 IU daily significantly reduced the risk of falling compared with a placebo in a dose-stratified analysis of the effect of 5 months of vitamin D supplementation on fall risk (72% lower incidence rate ratio; rate ratio, 0.28; 95% CI, 0.10–0.75). **Lower doses of vitamin D, however, did not significantly change the rate of fall incidence compared with placebo.** (Broe et al, 2007)

A 2004 review of 12 randomized, controlled trials studying the effect of vitamin D supplementation on fall risk among both nursing home residents and community dwellers found a small benefit of supplementation on fall risk, an effect that was also shown in a review of randomized, controlled trials with strict inclusion criteria, which included 1,237 men and women with a mean age of 70 years and supplementation for 2 months to 3 years. The pooled results showed a significant 22% decrease in fall risk among those treated with vitamin D versus placebo or calcium only. **The number needed to treat from the pooled results was 15 to prevent 1 person from falling**. (Bischoff_Ferrari et al, 2004)

Assessing vitamin D levels in a population at high risk for falling and supplementing with 800 to 1000 IU daily of vitamin D should be a part of any fall prevention program.

Vitamin D and Cancer

Both observational studies in humans and animal models support that vitamin D has a beneficial role in cancer prevention and survival. The mechanism of action is probably related to its role in the regulation of cell growth and differentiation.

In the 2006 Health Professionals Follow-Up study (a cohort study of 1095 men), each increment in 25(OH)D level of 25mmol/L was associated with a 17% reduction of total cancer cases. (Giovannucci et al, 2006)

However, the National Health and Nutrition Examination Survey of 16,818 men and women did not find a relationship between total cancer mortality and vitamin D level. There was an inverse relationship between vitamin D level and colorectal cancer, however. In this study, serum 25(OH)D levels of ≥80 nmol/L conferred a 72% reduction in risk of colorectal cancer compared with a level lower than 50 nmol/L. (Freedman et al, 2007)

A 2006 meta-analysis of 63 observational studies looked at the relationship between vitamin D levels and cancer incidence and mortality. **Twenty of the 30 studies looking at vitamin D and colon cancer showed that people with higher vitamin D levels had either a lower incidence of colon cancer or decreased mortality. Similarly, 9 of the 13 studies about breast cancer and 13 of the 26 studies about prostate cancer showed beneficial effects of vitamin D levels on cancer incidence or mortality** (some of the studies included more than one type of cancer). (Garland et al, 2006)

A 2007 population-based randomized, control trial found that **postmenopausal women who were supplemented with calcium and vitamin D had a reduced risk of cancer after the first year of treatment.** (Lappe et al, 2007)

There was not a group that was supplemented with vitamin D alone.

Vitamin D and Multiple Sclerosis

Multiple sclerosis (MS) is a neurodegenerative, T lymphocyte-mediated, autoimmune disease of uncertain etiology. Although genetic susceptibility may be involved, epidemiologic studies suggest environmental influence because **the development of MS correlates most strongly with rising latitude in both the northern and southern hemispheres**.

Migration studies show that risk can be modified at an early age from both low to high and high to low prevalence rates. **Exposure to sun in early childhood is associated with reduced risk of developing MS** and population-based studies about MS in Canada have also shown that birth timing is a risk factor for MS because there are statistically significantly fewer patients with MS born in November and more born in May compared with controls. A birth-timing association suggests that seasonality and sunlight exposure may also have an effect on the developing fetus in utero.

Several studies have shown that vitamin D affects the growth and differentiation of immune-modulator cells such as macrophages, dendritic cells, T cells, and B cells. (Holick, 2004) (Adorini, Penna, 2008)

This immune-modulatory effect has implications for a variety of autoimmune diseases including rheumatoid arthritis, systemic lupus erythematosous, type I DM, inflammatory bowel disease, and MS.

Despite the wealth of epidemiologic studies supporting a relationship between vitamin D and MS in humans, data showing a link between serum vitamin D levels and MS are only beginning to emerge. One prospective, nested, case-control study examined the serum samples of 7 million military veterans and compared serum samples of 257 MS patients before diagnosis with those of matched controls.

An inverse relationship between vitamin D levels and MS risk was found, particularly for vitamin D levels measured in patients younger than 20. Another case-control study compared the serum vitamin D levels of 103 MS patients with 110 controls and found that **for every 10-nmol/L increase of serum 25(OH)D level the odds of MS was reduced by 19% in women, suggesting a "protective" effect of higher vitamin D levels**. (Kragt et al, 2009)

In addition, a negative correlation was found between Expanded Disability Status Scale scores among female MS patients and 25(OH)D levels. Several other studies have supported the finding that **lower levels of vitamin D in MS patients are associated with more severe disability**. Lower levels during relapses have also been reported in patients with relapse-remitting MS.

The potential effects of oral vitamin D intake have been observed in several different ways. A Norwegian case-control study found that **fish and cod liver oil have a protective effect against the development of MS**. A large observational study in the United States that followed 2 large cohorts of women—the Nurses' Health Study (92,253 women followed from 1980 to 2000) and the Nurses' Health Study II (95,310 women followed from 1991 to 2001)—found that **vitamin D supplementation in the form of a multivitamin seemed to lower their MS risk by 40%.** (Munger et al, 2004)

However, several methodological weaknesses in study design made the results inconclusive. (Smolders et al, 2008)

Despite the overwhelming amount of data describing the association between vitamin D and MS, there is a paucity of research describing the benefit of vitamin D supplementation to these patients. One small safety study of 12 patients taking 1000 µg per day (40,000 IU) of vitamin D for 28 weeks showed a decline in the number of gadolinium-enhancing lesions on magnetic resonance imaging per patient; this led to a 25(OH) D serum concentration of 386 nmol/L (158 ng/mL) without causing hypercalcemia, hypercalciuria, or other complication.

Vitamin D and Cognition

Observational studies have shown that **people with Alzheimer dementia have lower vitamin D levels than do matched controls without dementia.** (Buell et al, 2008)

The biological plausibility of this relationship includes **vitamin D's antioxidative effects** and the presence of vitamin D receptors in the hippocampus, which has been seen in rats and humans. (Buell et al, 2008)

A cross-sectional study of 225 outpatients diagnosed with Alzheimer disease found a correlation between vitamin D levels (but not other vitamin levels) and their score on a Mini Mental Status Examination. (Oudshoom et al, 2008)

Vitamin D and Chronic Pain

Because of the important role vitamin D plays in bone homeostasis, some have questioned whether vitamin D deficiency may also correlate with chronic pain syndromes, including chronic low back pain. Several case series and observational studies have suggested that vitamin D inadequacy may represent a source of nociception and impaired neuromuscular functioning among patients with chronic pain.

The data to support this conclusion are **mixed**. A recent 2009 review of 22 relevant studies **found no convincing link between prevalence and latitude and no association between serum levels of 25-OH vitamin D in chronic pain patients and controls.** Interestingly, though, there was a contrast in treatment effects between randomized, double-blind trials that minimized bias and those with studies known to be subject to bias. **In those that blinded the vitamin D therapy, only 10% of patients were in trials showing a benefit of vitamin D treatment, whereas among those who did not blind the treatment, 93% were in trials showing a benefit of vitamin D supplementation.** (Straube et al, 2009)

A second review examined the role of vitamin deficiency in patients from outpatient and inpatient rehab units. Fifty-one articles were reviewed and **a direct correlation was noted between vitamin D deficiency and musculoskeletal pain.**

Treatment of vitamin D deficiency produced an increase in muscle strength and a marked decrease in back and lower-limb pain within 6 months.

Although these data were suggestive of a link between vitamin D and pain, **the available evidence does not imply causality.** The verdict on this topic **will remain undecided** until this is evaluated by double-blind, randomized, controlled trials stratified by baseline vitamin D level with defined treatments and comparison placebo groups.

Testing for Vitamin D Deficiency

There are many causes of vitamin D deficiency and despite growing attention to this deficiency, **there are no established guidelines to help clinicians decide which patients warrant screening laboratory testing for vitamin D deficiency.** The US Preventive Services Task Force does not comment for or against routine screening for vitamin D deficiency. One approach is to consider serum testing in patients at high risk for vitamin D deficiency but treating without testing those at lower risk.

A 2005 Australian working group issued a position statement itemizing groups of people **at risk for vitamin D deficiency**.

The risk groups include:

(1) older people in low- and high-level residential care;

(2) older people admitted to hospital;

(3) patients with hip fracture;

(4) dark-skinned women (particularly if veiled); and

(5) mothers of infants with rickets (particularly if dark-skinned or veiled). (Working group, 2005)

If electing to test vitamin D status, serum 25-hydroxyvitamin D is the accepted biomarker.

Although 1,25-OH-D is the active circulating form of vitamin D, measuring this level is not helpful because it is quickly and tightly regulated by the kidney. True deficiency would be evident only by measuring 25-OH-D. Of note, questions have been raised regarding the need for standardization of assays. (Binkley et al, 2004)

A large laboratory (Quest Diagnostics) recently reported the possibility of thousands of incorrect vitamin D level results. (Pollack, 2009)

Sunlight exposure questionnaires are imprecise and are not currently recommended.

Controversy exists regarding the optimum level of serum 25-hydroxyvitamin D in a healthy population. Most experts agree that serum vitamin D levels <20 ng/mL represent deficiency. However, some experts recommend aiming for a higher minimum target level of 30 ng/mL of 25-hydroxyvitamin D in a healthy population.

Vitamin D intoxication can occur when serum levels are greater than 150 ng/mL. Symptoms of hypervitaminosis D include fatigue, nausea, vomiting, and weakness probably caused by the resultant hypercalcemia. Of note, sun exposure alone cannot lead to vitamin D intoxication as excess vitamin D_3 is destroyed by sunlight.

More Vitamin D Recommended for Kids 3-13-09

The American Academy of Pediatrics has doubled the recommended daily dose of vitamin D for children and teens up to 400 units per day, which is equivalent to drinking four cups of milk.

Estimates are that 60,000 cases of colon cancer and 85,000 cases of breast cancer could be prevented every year in the U.S. for those who maintain a vitamin D level of at least 55 ng/mL.

Vitamin D improves muscle strength and is necessary for the effective absorption of dietary calcium, which becomes deposited in bones and teeth. Individual vitamin D requirements depend on your age and your amount of sunlight exposure.

New research indicates that teens with the lowest vitamin D levels are more than twice as likely to have high blood pressure and high blood sugar, which sets them up for hypertension and diabetes. Teens in the study were also four times more likely to have a dangerous condition called "metabolic syndrome."

However, **the Johns Hopkins Bloomberg School of Public Health reminds us that these are "strong associations" and not proof of causality.** Experts say that getting about 15 minutes of sunlight exposure a few times a week is generally enough and point out that vitamin D is found in fatty fish like salmon and is added to milk.

Other studies suggest that it helps lower blood pressure, reduces inflammation and boosts the immune system. Additionally, vitamin D3 supplementation has been arguably linked to lower risks of cancer, arthritis, tuberculosis and diabetes.

Patients with higher vitamin D3 levels appear to have lower rates of breast, colon, ovarian, prostate, pancreatic and lymphomatous cancers. My research indicates that vitamin D3 has such wide ranging beneficial effects because of its strong prooxidant activity (www.iwillfindthecure.org).

We welcome medical news which offers preventative measures for major health problems such as hypertension, cancer and diabetes.

More importantly, it has minimal downside and adverse effects, although over dosage can carry health hazards. As always, check with your physician regarding questions. Please remember, "Treat your body like it belongs to you."

UK Experts call for clarity prescribing and dispensing of vitamin D

June 13, 2014

Vitamin D is a steroid vitamin, a group of fat-soluble prohormones, which encourages the absorption and metabolism of calcium and phosphorous.

Leading independent specialists with an interest in vitamin D have called on **NICE** (National Institute for Health and Care Excellence) to make clear the importance of regulated vitamin D products licensed by the MHRA (i.e., either prescription only medicines (POMs), pharmacy medicines (P) or general sales list (GSL) in its forthcoming public health guideline 'Vitamin D: implementation of existing guidance to prevent deficiency'. (NICE, 2014) (NICE http://www.nice.org.uk/nicemedia/live/13795/67630/67630.pdf)

They fear that unless the guideline makes clear that only licensed vitamin D products should be recommended, prescribed and dispensed, the large and vulnerable group whom the UK CMOs stipulate should be given vitamin D to prevent deficiency could be at risk of receiving either a sub-therapeutic or an excessive dose.

Vitamin D, a sterol hormone, is essential for skeletal growth and bone health. Vitamin D deficiency is a serious and increasing UK public health priority, with the latest data from the National Diet & Nutrition Survey show that **around 20% of adults in the UK are deficient.** (FSA, 2012)

One of the clinical consequences of Vitamin D deficiency in adults is osteomalacia. (NOS, 2013)

In children, deficiency can result in rickets, and there is evidence to show that this condition is re-emerging in the UK. (Lowdon, 2011)

Dr Michael Stone, Director of Bone Research, University Hospital, Llandough said: "NICE has a duty to ensure that prescribers and dispensing pharmacists are aware that licenced vitamin D products are available, safe and cost effective. There is no justification for unlicensed products purporting to be medicines to be available on prescription and we call on NICE to accept our recommendation in its final guideline due out in the Autumn".

The Medicines and Healthcare Products Regulatory Agency, the General Medical Council and the Royal Pharmaceutical Society all clearly state that where there is an available licensed medicine, it should be prescribed and dispensed in preference to an unlicensed product purporting to be a medicine, such as a food supplement. Not doing so raises potential medico-legal issues for the prescriber and the dispensing pharmacist.

Yet, Prescription Cost Analysis data shows that the exponential increase in the use of vitamin D products on the NHS in recent years, has been driven by the dispensing of unlicensed products purporting to be medicines.

Data comparing similarly formulated preparations reveals, that, in general, licensed preparations are almost 50% less expensive per 1,000 international units supplied.

Dr Sally Hope, previously a GP Principal for 26 years, now Clinical Assistant in metabolic bone in Oxford said: "I am concerned that the current draft guideline does not acknowledge the difference between medicines licensed by the MHRA and products purporting to be medicines. In its current form, this guideline has the potential to cause confusion among prescribers, dispensing pharmacists and the general public. There are risks for prescribers if prescriptions are filled using unlicensed products."

Dr Brian Curwain, independent pharmaceutical consultant commented: "Food supplements are variable in their composition, both in terms of the active ingredient and potentially allergenic excipients, colours etc, that they contain. It is important that NICE acknowledges that there are greater risks to health professionals in terms of their legal responsibility in supplying food supplements than in licensed vitamin D medicines."

The public consultation on the draft guidance closes on 24 June and final guidance is expected in November 2014.

Vitamin D insufficiency is highest among people who are elderly, institutionalized, or hospitalized.

In the United States, 60% of nursing home residents and 57% of hospitalized patients were found to be vitamin D deficient. A study from Boston determined that nearly two thirds of healthy, young adults in Boston were vitamin D insufficient at the end of winter.

Inadequate exposure to sunlight causes a deficiency in cutaneously synthesized vitamin D. **Diseases associated with vitamin D malabsorption include celiac sprue, short bowel syndrome, and cystic fibrosis.**

Breast milk has only minimal amounts of vitamin D. The American Academy of Pediatrics recommends vitamin D supplementation starting at age 2 months for infants fed exclusively with breast milk.

Vitamin D deficiency is often a silent disease. Severe vitamin D deficiency in children can present as bowing of the legs from rickets. In adults with a severe vitamin D deficiency, the examination can reveal periosteal bone pain. This is best detected using firm pressure on the sternal bone or tibia.

A 25(OH)D level of less than 32 ng/mL is considered vitamin D insufficient.

A 25(OH)D level of less than 20 ng/mL has been used to define vitamin D deficiency.

Intestinal calcium absorption is optimized at levels of more than 32 ng/mL. Parathyroid hormone levels start to rise at 25(OH)D levels less than 31 ng/mL, which is another marker for vitamin D insufficiency.

Individuals who do not have exposure to sunlight are at risk for vitamin D deficiency if they do not ingest adequate amounts of foods that contain vitamin D. However, **most dietary sources of vitamin D do not contain sufficient amounts of vitamin D to satisfy daily requirements.**

Foods thought to contain high amounts of vitamin D$_3$ include oily fish (e.g., salmon, mackerel, blue fish) as well as fortified milk and other dairy products.

Vegetables are not a good source of vitamin D.

Vitamin D deficiency generalities

http://www.vitamindcouncil.org/about-vitamin-d/am-i-deficient-in-vitamin-d/?gclid=CjgKEAjwwuqcBRCSuoivmlPnkwQSJACpqj3kxM uNf53MT4plXUXqAgnQBWp4XC0pqHaVJTn0GUi63_D_BwE#. Accessed 6-13-14.

For a number of reasons, many people aren't getting enough vitamin D to stay healthy. This is called vitamin D deficiency. You may not get enough vitamin D if:

- You don't get enough sunlight. Your body is usually able to get all the vitamin D it needs if you regularly expose enough bare skin to the sun. However, many people don't get enough sunlight because they spend a lot of time inside and because they use sunscreen. It's also difficult for some people to get enough vitamin D from the sun during the winter.

- You don't take supplements. It's very difficult to get enough vitamin D from the foods you eat alone.

- Your body needs more vitamin D than usual, for example if you're obese or pregnant.

There are some groups of people that are more likely to have vitamin D deficiency. **The following people are more likely to be lacking in vitamin D**:

- People with darker skin. The darker your skin the more sun you need to get the same amount of vitamin D as a fair-skinned person. For this reason, if you're Black, you're much more likely to have vitamin D deficiency that someone who is White.

- People who spend a lot of time indoors during the day. For example, if you're housebound, work nights or are in a hospital for a long time.

- People who cover their skin all of the time. For example, if you wear sunscreen or if your skin is covered with clothes.

- People that live in the North of the United States or Canada. This is because there are fewer hours of overhead sunlight the further away you are from the equator.

- Older people have thinner skin than younger people and this may mean that they can't produce as much vitamin D.

- Infants that are breastfed and aren't given a vitamin D supplement. If you're feeding your baby on breast milk alone, and you don't give your baby a vitamin D supplement or take a supplement yourself, your baby is more likely to be deficient in vitamin D.

- Pregnant women.

- People who are very overweight (obese).

Symptoms of vitamin D deficiency
The symptoms of vitamin D deficiency are sometimes vague and can **include tiredness and general aches and pains.** Some people may not have any symptoms at all.

If you have a severe vitamin D deficiency you may have pain in your bones and weakness, which may mean you have difficulty getting around. You may also have frequent infections. However, not everyone gets these symptoms.

If you think you may have vitamin D deficiency, you should see your physician, or have a blood test to check your vitamin D levels.

The way doctors measure if you're deficient in vitamin D is by testing your 25(OH)D level, but most doctors just call this a vitamin D test. Getting this blood test is the only accurate way to know if you're deficient or not.

(Holick, 2010) (Plum et al, 2010)

Vitamin D: Pros and Cons

This article by Jane Langille also gives a current balanced overview and appears with minimal modification.

In the last several years, there has been a flood of health **news about studies linking vitamin D deficiency with cancer, cardiovascular diseases, diabetes, metabolic disorders, depression, infectious diseases, autoimmune diseases, mortality and even autism.** A search on PubMed for vitamin D finds more than 1,400 papers listed from January to April 2014 alone.

As a result of this increased interest, some people are boosting their intake above the recommended dietary allowance hoping that extra vitamin D might help prevent, treat or cure a host of adverse disease conditions.

There currently is somewhat of a vitamin D craze in America.

Vitamin D supplementation is proven to be effective to help maintain good bone health, but can increasing intake above the current recommended dietary allowance really cure or prevent other health conditions?

Vitamin D and Arthritis

Here is an anecdotal case.

Dawn Hunter, a freelance editor based in Toronto, Ontario, takes 2,000 IU (international units) of vitamin D daily, even though some health guidelines call for a much smaller dose of 600 IU per day. "Every time I stop taking it, my levels just plummet," says Hunter, who has arthritis and says that she does not have the opportunity to get much natural sunshine.

Five years ago, Hunter found out she was severely deficient after her rheumatologist ordered a blood test. She addressed her deficiency by taking 4,000 IU daily for a year to boost her blood level from 14.8 ng/mL (nanograms per milliliter) and has been maintaining her level at 30.4 ng/mL with a daily dose of 2,000 IU for the past 4 years. (The normal range is 30.0 to 74.0 ng/mL).

"When my vitamin D level increased, I noticed a small reduction in the general ache I had with my arthritis," notes Hunter. "My rheumatologist says there is some evidence that arthritis can progress faster in people who have low levels of vitamin D. I was just turning 40 when my arthritis was diagnosed, so managing progression is important to me."

Arthritis Update 9-2-13

Rheumatoid arthritis (rheumatoid disease) is a chronic (long lasting), progressive and disabling autoimmune disease that causes inflammation (swelling) and pain in the joints and the tissue around the joints.

Unlike the wear-and-tear damage of osteoarthritis, rheumatoid arthritis (RA) affects the lining of your joints, causing a painful swelling that can eventually result in bone erosion and joint deformity.

RA is an auto-immune disease, which is 2-3 times more common in women than men and usually begins after the age of forty and in the small joints. It is four times more common in smokers than non-smokers.

About 0.6% of the United States adult population has RA.

There is no evidence that physical and emotional effects or stress trigger the disease. The many negative findings suggest that either the trigger varies, or that it might be a chance event inherent with the immune response.

However, epidemiological studies have confirmed a potential association between RA and two herpes virus infections.

Vitamin D deficiency is common in those with RA and may be causally associated.

Some trials have found a decreased risk for RA with vitamin D supplementation while others have not.

Recent studies from the UK suggests that sulforaphane, a compound found in broccoli and other cruciferous vegetables such as cabbage and Brussels sprouts, could help fight osteoarthritis, the most common form of arthritis.

Sulforaphane is released when eating curciferous vegetables such as broccoli, cauliflower, brussels sprouts, kale, cabbage, bok choy or Chinese cabbage.

Osteoarthritis is a painful and often limiting joint disease affecting the hands, feet, spine, hips and knees in particular. According to the US

Centers for Disease Control and Prevention (CDC), the condition affects 27 million American adults.

Age and obesity are the most common contributors to osteoarthritis and there is currently no cure. The Department of Health and Human Services' recommends 150 minutes of moderate exercise per week and there was no increased risk of developing knee osteoarthritis with this regime.

According to JAMA, overweight and obese adults suffering from knee osteoarthritis may benefit more from combined intensive diet and exercise regimes, rather than undertaking diet or exercise regimes separately.

Combining diet and exercise also showed reduced knee pain, better function, faster walking speed and better physical health-related quality of life, compared with the exercise-only group.

Diet participants were required to follow a weekly meal plan, including up to two meal-replacement shakes a day and a meal between 500-750 kcal that was low in fat and high in vegetables.

We should try to exercise for 1 hour a day, 3 days a week (aerobic walking, 15- 30 minutes), strength training (20 minutes), and a cool-down, combined with a healthy fruit and vegetable diet.

Vitamin D is really a hormone

Vitamin D is actually a pro-hormone that is involved in many metabolic processes. Your body makes vitamin D from sunlight on your skin,.

Supplements come in two formats: **vitamin D2 (ergocalciferol)** and **vitamin D3 (cholecalciferol)**. Vitamin D2 is found naturally in sun-exposed mushrooms.

Vitamin D3 is the form made naturally in human skin and is **made from a cholesterol precursor** obtained from lanolin. It can be found in oil-rich fish like salmon, mackerel and herring.

There is some evidence that the D3 format is more bioavailable.

Vitamin D is fat-soluble, meaning that if you take too much, the excess is not excreted in urine.

In your body, your liver converts vitamin D from sunlight or supplements to 25-hydroxyvitamin D, [25(OH)D], the form that is measured in a blood test. The 25 (OH)D is then converted again, mostly in the kidneys, to the activated form of vitamin D, a hormone called **calcitriol (1,25-dihydroxyvitamin D).**

It's plausible that vitamin D may play a role in a host of other diseases and conditions such as cancer, cardiovascular disease and diabetes, because there are calcitriol receptors on nearly all tissues in the body.

Calcitriol plays a role in regulation of over 900 different genes. In cell culture and animal studies, researchers have found that **calcitriol is involved in cell differentiation, proliferation and inhibition, inflammation, and the synthesis and secretion of insulin.**

Calcitriol also has an impact on brain function and development. Two U.S. researchers recently proposed a mechanism to explain how calcitriol may be involved in the regulation of the production of serotonin, a brain chemical that is often out of balance in autistic children.

At first blush, it may seem hard to believe that vitamin D could be associated with so many different conditions. However, John J. Cannell, MD, Founder and Executive Director of the Vitamin D Council, says, "Many people are turned off by these claims and say it's impossible that one thing is involved in so many different disease processes, but they are unaware of the mechanism of vitamin D.

It (vitamin D) is actually a steroid hormone precursor that turns genes on and off. There are at least a thousand genes that are allegedly directly regulated by vitamin D."

Recent vitamin D studies

Here are some examples of recent studies that found a link between vitamin D and health conditions.

Cholesterol

Vitamin D may improve cholesterol numbers. A recent study analyzed data from 576 postmenopausal women who were part of the **National Institute of Health's Women's Health Initiative trial.** Women who took 400 IU of vitamin D plus 1,000 mg of calcium daily showed a significantly higher blood level of vitamin D after two years, compared to the control group who took a placebo. Interestingly, **those who had higher blood levels of vitamin D also had better lipid profiles, showing increased high-density ("good") cholesterol), decreased low-density ("bad") cholesterol and lower triglycerides**.

The researchers acknowledge that the sample size was small and their **findings are not conclusive** about how vitamin D affects cardiovascular health. However, given that these results were from blood work for women followed for several years, there is a relationship here that merits further research. The study was published in the March 2014 issue of Menopause.

Breast cancer

Patients with higher levels of vitamin D at the time of breast cancer diagnosis may live longer. A recent meta-analysis combined data from more than 4,500 breast cancer patients from 5 observational studies to see if higher vitamin D levels at the time of breast cancer diagnosis were associated with longer patient survival times.

Over a 9-year period, **patients in the group with the highest blood level of 25-dihydroxyvitamin D [25(OH)D], (the form of vitamin D measured in blood tests), at an average level of 30 ng/mL, had about half the fatality rate compared to those in the group with the lowest level of 17 ng/mL on average**.

In the paper, **researchers reported that other lab studies have shown that vitamin D has anticancer effects, arresting tumor growth in 3 critical phases of development**.

While these results are encouraging, the researchers caution that **a causal conclusion is not possible** and that a randomized controlled trial is needed to shed further light on the findings. The study was published in the March 2014 issue of Anticancer Research.

Risk of Mortality

Low vitamin D levels carry a greater risk of death.

In a large systematic review and meta-analysis published in the April 2014 issue of the British Medical Journal, researchers looked at the link between vitamin D and chronic diseases to assess mortality risk.

They combined data from several large databases of studies, including Medline, Embase and the Cochrane Library. **Low blood levels of vitamin D were associated with a greater risk of death from cardiovascular disease, cancer and other causes.**

Calculations showed that **each 10 ng/mL decline of 25(OH)D was associated with a 16% greater risk of mortality and that supplementation with vitamin D3 reduced mortality risk by 11%.**

Autism

Vitamin D may play a role in abnormal social behavior seen in people with autism spectrum disorder. Rhonda Patrick, PhD, and **Bruce Ames**, PhD, at the Children's Hospital Oakland Research Center (CHORI) in California, proposed a causal mechanism for how 3 brain hormones that influence social behavior — serotonin, oxytocin and vasopressin — are activated by vitamin D at the genetic level. These brain hormones are often out of balance in children with autism spectrum disorder. These researchers hypothesize (guessed) that the drop in adequate levels of vitamin D in the U.S. over the past few decades – due in part to increased use of sunscreens and more indoor work — may in part explain the increase in autism rates. The study was published in the February issue of The Journal of the Federation of American Societies for Experimental Biology.

Different views on the ideal level of vitamin D?

Almost 70% of the U.S. population has insufficient levels of 25(OH)D, when defined as less than 30 ng/mL, according to data combined from many studies.

The level of vitamin D in your body is measured by a blood test that measures **25-hydroxyvitamin D, [25(OH)D], the form of vitamin D that your body makes after converting what you receive from sunlight on skin, supplements or from some food sources, such as fortified milk and orange juice or from the flesh of fatty fish, including salmon, tuna and mackerel.**

The Vitamin D Council, a nonprofit organization based in California that works to educate the public about vitamin D, notes that there are several factors that affect how much vitamin D your body produces when your skin is exposed to sunlight. These factors include the time of year and time of day of exposure, where you live and the type of skin you have. You can request a blood test to check your vitamin D levels from your doctor, and the cost is usually covered in the U.S. if a doctor orders it with the right diagnostic code.

According to the Institute of Medicine (IOM), the current recommended dietary intake of 600 IU for adults under the age of 70 years and 800 IU for adults over 70 years is sufficient to meet the needs of 97.5% of healthy adults who have minimal sun exposure.

The IOM defines sufficiency of 25(OH)D as greater than 20 ng/mL. This recommendation was based on proven benefits for bone health, as the IOM did not find convincing evidence about causal outcomes with other health conditions.

The Vitamin D Council recommends a much higher daily intake of 5,000 IU to achieve a sufficiency level of 50 ng/mL.

Dr. Cannell says, "The Vitamin D Council arrived at a recommendation very simply — to reproduce natural vitamin D from sun exposure. We know that natural vitamin D levels for lifeguards and roofers and hunter/gatherers from modern-day Tanzania are about 50 ng/mL. Until all the studies are done and all the science is completed, the safest thing for you to do is to maintain a natural vitamin D level."

The IOM, however, noted a concern for attaining levels above 50 ng/ mL and **designated 4,000 IU daily as the tolerable upper intake limit**, with the caution that this is not to be interpreted as a target intake level. JoAnn E. Manson, MD, DrPH, Chief of Preventive Medicine at Brigham and Women's Hospital and Professor of Medicine at Harvard Medical School, was on the IOM Committee that developed the guidelines. She says, "There's still a pretty wide range of intake in the IOM guidelines. The recommended dietary allowance is what will meet the requirements for a very large majority of the population, 97.5% in the U.S. and Canada, but the IOM is also saying that **there is a risk of adverse events at intake levels above 4,000 IU per day.**"

Risks of too much vitamin D

How much is too much? **Observational studies suggest that shooting for blood levels above 50 ng/mL may be associated** with an increased risk of pancreatic cancer, cardiovascular disease and an increased risk of death.

Dr. Manson says, "Some vitamin D is good, but more is not necessarily better. People should understand that there is limited research on long-term intakes above 2,000 IU daily. If they are regularly taking 3,000-4,000 IU per day, even if those levels may not have been linked to adverse events, we do not know if the benefits outweigh the risks long-term because we don't have the evidence."

Massive doses of 10,000 IU daily or more can put you at risk of developing high calcium levels in the blood, or in the urine, which could cause calcification of blood vessels, kidney problems and kidney stones, especially if calcium intake is also high.

Dr. Manson advises that it's important to distinguish between public health guidelines and medical situations where individual patients actually need more vitamin D, such as those who have bone health problems, malabsorption or who are on medications that may interfere with the metabolism of vitamin D. For example, **steroid drugs like prednisone, weight loss drugs like orlistat (Alli) and the cholesterol-lowering drug cholestyramine (Questran) can reduce the absorption of vitamin D.**

The National Institute of Health (NIH) identifies a number of interactions of moderate concern, including with the cholesterol-lowering statin Lipitor: "**Atorvastatin (Lipitor):** Vitamin D might decrease the amount of atorvastatin (Lipitor) that enters the body. This might decrease how well atorvastatin (Lipitor) works."

While there may be some situations that warrant higher doses of vitamin D, Dr. Manson cautions against taking mega-doses of the "sunshine" vitamin. "Clinicians still have latitude to make individualized recommendations for higher amounts for their patients, but the public health guidelines are saying that most of the population should not be taking high doses or getting blood screening tests regularly because there is no evidence to support that," says Dr. Manson

New evidence on the horizon

Experts are hoping a comprehensive trial underway called VITAL (VITamin D and OmegA-3 TriaL) will reveal the true health benefits of vitamin D. Dr. Manson is lead investigator for this large-scale U.S. study among 10,000 adult women over 55 and 10,000 men over 50. She and her colleague, Julie Buring, DSc, are investigating if taking daily doses of 2,000 IU of vitamin D or a supplement of omega-3 fatty acids (Omacor fish oil, 1 gram) can reduce the risk of developing cancer, heart disease and stroke in healthy people with no history of these diseases.

The study is a randomized, double-blind, placebo-controlled trial where the test groups and the comparison groups will have a large enough difference in vitamin D levels to see if there is a meaningful difference in health outcomes. The study began in 2008 and is collecting data over an average of 5 years. The National Cancer Institute and the National Heart, Lung and Blood Institute are primary sponsors for the VITAL Study and final results are expected in late 2017.

Right now, the excitement about vitamin D is focused on the promise it offers in helping with a host of health conditions beyond bone health. **"The enthusiasm is definitely outpacing the evidence,"** notes Dr. Manson.

"Although we know that vitamin D deficiency needs treatment, **there is a disconnect between the observational studies that have linked low vitamin D to nearly every known health condition and the randomized trials of high-dose vitamin D supplements that have been largely disappointing to date**.

We do need the large-scale randomized trials, though, to test rigorously whether supplementation above the recommended dietary allowance confers greater health benefits."

Vitamin D3 circa 2007

There is Good News and bad news for Vitamin D3

In 2007, Canadian researchers reported that children, later diagnosed with multiple sclerosis, had far lower levels of vitamin D than other youngsters and this was the first study to show links between the "sunshine" vitamin and a childhood disease, other than rickets.

Multiple sclerosis is a nervous system disease caused by damage to the myelin sheath that protects nerve cells and it affects 2.5 million people globally. Vitamin D is necessary for the effective absorption of dietary calcium, which becomes deposited in bones and teeth.

Your individual requirements depend on your age, the amount of sunlight exposure you get, liver and kidney function and medical conditions. **Generally, the recommended amount has been 400 IU a day for people ages 51 to 70, but that amount is increasing.**

For those over age 70, the recommendation was 600 IU a day but, in addition to modest sun exposure, adults can take up to 2,000 IU of vitamin D per day, which is the "tolerable upper intake level" set by U.S. health officials.

More than 2,000 IU a day can cause toxicity problems including excessive urination, high blood pressure, nausea, weight loss, fatigue, calcium deposits in soft tissues (kidney stones) and kidney damage. Vitamin D3 is found in fatty fish like salmon and is added to milk and other foods. Data suggests it helps lower blood pressure, reduces inflammation and boosts the immune system.

High doses of vitamin D3 have been linked to lower risks of cancer, arthritis, tuberculosis and diabetes. Lower rates of breast, colon, ovarian, prostate, pancreatic and lymphomatous cancers are seen in patients with higher vitamin D3 levels and vitamin D3 helps prevent cancer cells from growing and spreading.

We must rely on safe means of protecting ourselves from disease and the judicious intake of vitamin D3 seems to be on target. The D3 form appears to be most effective and it is readily available and inexpensive. However, do not assume that "more is always better." Use good common sense, exercise, eat fresh fruits and vegetables and avoid unnecessary pharmaceuticals whenever possible.

Vitamin D: Up to 800-1,000 IU daily (less if you live in a year-round warm climate and get 15 minutes of unblocked sun every day). Get it from a separate pill or with calcium. Vitamin D and calcium go hand in hand.

It is hard to consume 600 IUs of vitamin D from food alone. A cup of D-fortified milk or orange juice has about 100 IUs. The best sources may be fatty fish — some servings of salmon can provide about a day's supply. Other good sources are D-fortified cereals.

However, a study on 11-30-10 by the Institute of Medicine recommends: "Most people in the U.S. and Canada — from age 1 to age 70 — need to consume no more than 600 international units of vitamin D a day to maintain health, the report found. People in their 70s and older need as much as 800 IUs. The report set those levels as the "recommended dietary allowance" for vitamin D."

A National Cancer Institute study last summer was the latest to report no cancer protection from vitamin D and the possibility of an increased risk of pancreatic cancer in people with the very highest D levels.

Super-high doses, above 10,000 IUs a day, are known to cause kidney damage.

Dr. Joann Manson of Harvard Medical School, who co-authored the Institute of Medicine's report, pointed to history's cautionary tales: **"A list of other supplements — vitamins C and E and beta carotene — plus menopause hormone pills that once were believed to prevent cancer or heart disease didn't pan out, and sometimes caused harm, when put to rigorous testing."**

As for calcium, the report recommended already accepted levels to go along with your daily D — about 1,000 milligrams of calcium a day for most adults, 700 to 1,000 mg for young children, and 1,300 mg for teenagers and menopausal women. Too much can cause kidney stones; the report said that risk increases once people pass 2,000 mg a day.

Calcium: Up to 1,000 mg total from food and supplements. If you don't eat 3 servings of milk/dairy, take the equivalent in a supplement that contains vitamin D3.

Vitamin D deficiency doubles the risk of fatal stroke in whites but not in blacks

A November, 2010 report in the Los Angeles Times said **vitamin D deficiency doubles the risk of fatal strokes in whites, but has no effect on the risk in blacks**, even though blacks are more likely to have vitamin D deficiencies and are 65% more likely to die from strokes, researchers said. The results were puzzling, said Dr. Erin Michos of the Johns Hopkins School of Medicine in Baltimore. "We thought maybe the lower vitamin D levels might actually explain why blacks have higher risks for strokes," she said.

Stroke is the third leading cause of death in the United States, killing more than 140,000 Americans annually and permanently disabling more than half a million.

Michos and her colleagues analyzed health records of 7,981 black and white adults who participated in the Third National Health and Nutrition Examination Survey of Americans, conducted between 1988 and 1994, following the participants for a median of 14 years. They reported at a Chicago meeting of the American Heart Assn. that, among the participants, **6.6% of whites and 32.3% of blacks had severely low levels of vitamin D in their blood, classified as levels below 15 nanograms per milliliter**.

During the period of the study, 116 whites and 60 blacks died of stroke. Accounting for age and other risk factors, **blacks were 65% more likely to suffer a stroke**.

Higher levels of diabetes and hypertension probably account for some of the increased risk, but not this much, Michos said. "Something else is surely behind this problem. However, don't blame vitamin D deficits."

The lack of sensitivity to low levels of vitamin D may be an adaptation to historic low levels associated with the sun-blocking effects of skin pigments, she added. The blacks in the study also had fewer incidents of bone fracture and greater overall bone density than whites. "In blacks, we may not need to raise vitamin D levels to the same level as in whites to minimize their risk of stroke," she concluded

SECTION TWO

NEGATIVE STUDIES: DISCREDITING SCIENCE

Thoughts on vitamin D deficiency

Vitamin D is made by the body under the skin when it is exposed to sunlight. A deficiency can cause problems when there is not enough of the vitamin to properly absorb the required levels of calcium and phosphate.

Mild to moderate vitamin D deficiency can lead to bone pain and weakening of the bones – osteoporosis – which increases the risk of fractures.

More severe levels of deficiency can lead to the development of rickets in children and osteomalacia in adults.
And a 2010 British Medical Journal clinical review found that vitamin D deficiency can increase the risk of developing heart disease, bowel and breast cancer, multiple sclerosis and diabetes.

Professor Cedric Garland said:'Three years ago, the Institute of Medicine concluded that having a too-low blood level of vitamin D was hazardous. This study supports that conclusion, but goes one step further. The 20 nanograms per milliliter (ng/ml) blood level cutoff assumed from the IOM report was based solely on the association of low vitamin D with risk of bone disease.

Prof Randolph M. Howes MD,PhD

Vitamin D Blog: Ioannidis Paints Bleak Picture circa 2014

Published: Apr 7, 2014

By Kristina Fiore, Staff Writer, MedPage Today

There's no "highly convincing" evidence linking vitamin D and any outcome, even musculoskeletal benefits, according to famed research skeptic John Ioannidis and his colleagues.

In an umbrella review of 268 observational studies and meta-analyses published in *BMJ*, they turned up no clear ties between vitamin D intake and several diseases, although there may be associations with a selection of outcomes, they wrote.

Even though the vitamin has been associated with 137 outcomes in reports (including skeletal, malignant, cardiovascular, autoimmune, infectious, metabolic and other diseases), the researchers found only 10 had been well studied.

The only evidence of benefit appeared to be for birth weight and the mother's vitamin D status; there were "probable" associations with a few other outcomes -- dental caries in children, maternal vitamin D levels at term, and parathyroid hormone levels in dialysis patients -- but better-designed trials are needed to draw firmer conclusions, they wrote.

They said **the findings cast doubt on vitamin D for osteoporosis, and it "might not be as essential as previously thought in maintaining bone mineral density."**

In a second study in the same issue of the journal, Rajiv Chowdhury and colleagues looked at 73 cohort studies and 22 randomized controlled trials to assess the link between vitamin D and chronic diseases.

They did find that **low circulating levels of the vitamin were associated with increased risk of death from cardiovascular disease, cancer, and other causes, and that supplementation with vitamin D3 cut mortality risk by 11% (but supplementation with vitamin D2 did not).**

Chowdhury and colleagues warned, however, that more study would be needed to determine the optimal dose of vitamin D3.

70

Naveed Sattar, MD, PhD, and Paul Welsh, PhD, of Glasgow University in Scotland, wrote in an accompanying editorial that the latter study was limited by observational data and that the results aren't a "green light for widespread D3 supplementation."

They warned that doctors should avoid "costly measurement" of vitamin D levels in healthy patients -- at least in those who don't have bone disease.

Vitamin D Blog: Review Draws Flood of Letters to Journal

Published: Apr 9, 2014 | Updated: Apr 9, 2014

By Kristina Fiore, Staff Writer, MedPage Today

An endocrinology journal received a deluge of letters regarding a systematic review that found supplementation for vitamin D deficiency doesn't appear to reduce chronic disease risk.

Although some of the letters were positive, many took issue with the study, and author Philippe Autier, MD, MPH, of the International Prevention Research Institute in Lyon, France, and colleagues, issued a reply in the April issue of *The Lancet Diabetes & Endocrinology*.

Among the top names in vitamin D research critiquing the piece was Michael Holick, MD, PhD, of Boston University, who along with William Grant, PhD, of the Sunlight, Nutrition, and Health Research Center in San Francisco, said that an assessment based on the medical model "is not necessarily appropriate for natural compounds."

Autier and colleagues responded that vitamin D is indeed a drug, and that "many drugs are natural" and their efficacy is tested in randomized trials -- such as is the case with insulin.

Holick and Grant also "missed the crucial point" that despite low serum concentrations of active vitamin D, supplementation couldn't increase those levels "most likely because of deregulation of vitamin D metabolism associated with inflammation," Autier and colleagues wrote.

Declan Naughton, PhD, and Andrea Petroczi, PhD, both of Kingston University in London, England, contended that the full range of vitamin D metabolites needs to be considered, via tools that accurately measure several forms of vitamin D.

Prof Randolph M. Howes MD,PhD

"It is premature to come to association-based conclusions about such a complex set of metabolites until investigations capture the roles of several forms and supplementation with several forms," they wrote.

But Autier and colleagues wrote that it's unlikely the relevant vitamin D form hasn't been found during 50 years' worth of basic science and animal studies.

Several of the letters lamented the lack of study around the difference between vitamin D and solar radiation in terms of health effects.

"We are disappointed that the review ... omitted geographical evidence suggesting that increased levels of solar UV radiation ... is associated with a substantially reduced incidence of many diseases," wrote Cedric Garland, PhD, of the University of California San Diego.

Martin Feelisch, PhD, of the University of Southampton in England, and colleagues noted that **the "sun seems beneficial to health via a mechanism of action unrelated to vitamin D."**

Helen Macdonald, PhD, of the University of Aberdeen in Scotland, and colleagues acknowledged that the study may lead to others questioning the benefits of vitamin D: "We hope the results will not lead to years of debate, as happened with the Women's Health Initiative."

"We should be mindful that individuals who are most deficient in vitamin D are the ones most likely to benefit from supplementation," they wrote, "and exercise caution when extrapolating to the general population."

Vitamin D Blog: D Has No Effect on Depression

Published: Mar 20, 2014

By Kristina Fiore, Staff Writer, MedPage Today

Depressed patients won't get any relief from vitamin D supplementation, a new meta-analysis found.

In a review of seven trials totaling nearly 3,200 patients, the vitamin had no significant effect on depressive symptoms

overall, Jonathan Shaffer, PhD, of Columbia University Medical Center, in New York City, and colleagues reported in *Psychosomatic Medicine*.

However, when looking specifically at patients who had clinically significant depressive symptoms or depressive disorder, the researchers found that there did appear to be a moderately significant effect of vitamin D supplementation on symptoms.

In a press release, the researchers noted that further work should be done on whether vitamin D adds to improvements when patients are also on antidepressants.

They also noted that supplementation may work when depressed patients have an actual deficiency in vitamin D, but more studies are needed.

Vitamin D Fails to Ease Winter Coughs and Colds

February 21, 2014

"A randomized, placebo-controlled trial has found that **vitamin D and calcium, whatever their other benefits may be, have no effect on upper respiratory tract infections**." It is based on a four year study with 759 people via The New York Times.

Supplementation with 1000 IU/day vitamin D_3 did not significantly reduce the incidence or duration of URTI in adults with a baseline serum 25-hydroxyvitamin D level ≥12 ng/mL.

Original study can be found here: Clinical Infectious Disease Journal. Written By Nicholas Bakalar. Published on Dec. 2, 2013. (Rees et al, 2013)

Vitamin D Blog: D's Role in Weight Loss

Published: Mar 17, 2014

By Kristina Fiore, Staff Writer, MedPage Today

Simply supplementing vitamin D as part of a dietary intervention won't necessarily aid weight loss, unless patients actually

73

achieve levels of 25 (OH)D of 32 ng/mL or more. (Mason et al, 2014)

Those are the findings from a year-long **randomized controlled trial in 218 overweight and obese women with vitamin D insufficiency,** published in the *American Journal of Clinical Nutrition.*

Anne McTiernan, MD, PhD, of the Fred Hutchinson Cancer Research Center in Seattle, and colleagues randomized the women, all of whom were given a dietary intervention, to either 2,000 IU oral vitamin D3 daily or placebo.

Although there were no differences between groups by the end of the study in terms of weight loss or other metabolic parameters, they found that **within the vitamin D group, those who had achieved sufficiency lost significantly more weight than those who didn't (8.8 lbs versus 5.6 lbs, *P*=0.05).**

These women also had greater losses in waist circumference and body fat, McTiernan and colleagues reported.

It's still not clear exactly how vitamin D is involved in obesity. There's no way to tell if becoming vitamin D sufficient causes further weight loss, or if better weight loss led to improvements in vitamin D status.

But McTiernan and colleagues wrote that their study can help inform future trials that may be able to detect greater effects -- and can further tease those effects out -- if clinicians individualize supplementation so that more patients become vitamin D replete.

Vitamin D Blog: Anaphylaxis Tied to D Status?

Published: Mar 21, 2014

By Kristina Fiore, Staff Writer, MedPage Today
Researchers have found that **anaphylaxis may vary with exposure to sunlight** -- a marker of vitamin D status -- by looking at hospital admissions in Chile, a country that spans nearly 40° of latitude.

Rodrigo Hoyos-Bachiloglu, MD, of Pontificia Universidad Catolica de Chile in Santiago, and colleagues **found higher rates of admissions for anaphylaxis in more southern regions of the South**

American country, reporting their findings online in Pediatric Allergy and Immunology.

They studied about 2,300 anaphylaxis admissions from Chile's hospital discharge database between 2001 and 2010, and matched them up with latitude and solar radiation levels, proxies of vitamin D status.

There was a "**strong north-south increasing gradient of anaphylaxis admissions**" (P=0.01), and the southernmost region had the highest rate of admissions for the life-threatening condition, they reported.

They also found a significant association between solar radiation and anaphylaxis admissions (P=0.009).

Latitude was associated with food-induced but not drug-induced anaphylaxis -- which wasn't unexpected, they said, because of a stronger role of vitamin D deficiency in the pathogenesis of food-allergic reactions.

Additional analyses showed that **anaphylaxis admissions weren't associated with regional sociodemographic factors like poverty, education, ethnicity, physician density, or being in a rural area.**

Vitamin D deficiency may be an etiological factor in the high anaphylaxis admission rates found in southern Chile, they concluded.

Vitamin D Ineffective In Treating Asthma

In asthma and other diseases, vitamin D insufficiency is associated with adverse outcomes. It is not known if supplementing inhaled corticosteroids with oral vitamin D_3 improves outcomes in patients with asthma and vitamin D insufficiency.

Objective To evaluate if vitamin D supplementation would improve the clinical efficacy of inhaled corticosteroids in patients with symptomatic asthma and lower vitamin D levels.

Design, Setting, and Participants The VIDA (Vitamin D Add-on Therapy Enhances Corticosteroid Responsiveness in Asthma) randomized, double-blind, parallel, placebo-controlled trial studying adult patients with symptomatic asthma and a serum 25-hydroxyvitamin D level of less than 30 ng/mL was conducted across 9 academic US medical centers in the National Heart, Lung, and Blood Institute's AsthmaNet network, with enrollment starting in April 2011 and follow-up complete by January 2014. After a run-in period that included treatment with an inhaled corticosteroid, 408 patients were randomized.

Interventions Oral vitamin D_3 (100 000 IU once, then 4000 IU/d for 28 weeks; n = 201) or placebo (n = 207) was added to inhaled ciclesonide (320 µg/d). If asthma control was achieved after 12 weeks, ciclesonide was tapered to 160 µg/d for 8 weeks, then to 80 µg/d for 8 weeks if asthma control was maintained.

Main Outcomes and Measures The primary outcome was time to first asthma treatment failure (a composite outcome of decline in lung function and increases in use of β-agonists, systemic corticosteroids, and health care).

Results Treatment with vitamin D_3 did not alter the rate of first treatment failure during 28 weeks (28% with vitamin D_3 vs 29% with placebo; adjusted hazard ratio, 0.9. Of 14 prespecified secondary outcomes, 9 were analyzed, including asthma exacerbation; of those 9, **the only statistically significant outcome was a small difference in the overall dose of ciclesonide required to maintain asthma control** (111.3 µg/d in the vitamin D_3 group vs 126.2 µg/d in the placebo group; difference of 14.9 µg/d.

Conclusions and Relevance Vitamin D_3 did not reduce the rate of first treatment failure or exacerbation in adults with persistent asthma and vitamin D insufficiency. These findings do not support a strategy of therapeutic vitamin D_3 supplementation in patients with symptomatic asthma. (Castro et al, VIDA Trial, 2014) a randomized, double-blind, parallel, placebo-controlled trial.

There was also no significant reduction in the secondary end points related to asthma control, airway function, quality of life, or airway inflammation. (Castro et al, VIDA Trial, 2014) a randomized, double-blind, parallel, placebo-controlled trial.

Now, for the really bad news.

On December 1, 2010 the following study was released: **Vitamin D studies "inconsistent."**

After reviewing about 1,000 studies on the supposed links between low vitamin D levels and higher risk of serious diseases, a panel of US and Canadian doctors concluded that they showed inconsistent results, sometimes due to shoddy research methods. **The only sure benefit of the combination of calcium and vitamin D is bone health.**

The experts also issued **new guidelines**, the first since 1997, for North Americans, saying **people should take between 700 and 1,300 milligrams of calcium and anywhere from 600 to 800 international units of vitamin D each day.** The panel's establishment of new guidelines offer a more solid recommended daily dose than the 1997 approach of suggesting adequate intake (AI) amounts.

Glenville Jones, a Canadian doctor who was on the 14-member committee for the US-based Institute of Medicine, said, **"Vitamin D deficiency is quite rare in North Americans at this point in time."**

Humans need calcium to help clot blood and for proper functioning of muscles and nerves, and vitamin D is necessary for the body to absorb calcium. Inadequate calcium has been shown to lead to bone fractures and osteoporosis. And some populations are likely to need more Vitamin D than other groups, including breastfed babies, people with dark skin and those living in northern latitudes where daylight exposure is limited.

"Our dilemma is that there are mixed reports that are not all consistent," said Jones, who is a professor of biochemistry at Queens University in Kingston, Ontario. "Some of the studies are not well controlled," he said.

"We don't want to base public health recommendations upon a mixed conclusion where some studies say there is a benefit in cancer and other studies say they don't," he added.

The panel also set upper limits for both calcium (2,000 milligrams per day) and vitamin D (4,000 IUs per day), beyond which point risks such as kidney and tissue damage begin to mount. "Higher levels have not been shown to confer greater benefits, and in fact they have been linked to other health problems, challenging the concept that 'more is better,'" the report said.

Umbrella Review of Vitamin D

Vitamin D and multiple health outcomes: umbrella review of systematic reviews and meta-analyses of observational studies and randomized trials

Prof Randolph M. Howes MD,PhD

(Published 1 April 2014) (Vitamin D, Umbrella review, 2014)

Abstract

Investigators evaluated the breadth, validity, and presence of biases of the associations of vitamin D with diverse outcomes.

Design: Umbrella review of the evidence across systematic reviews and meta-analyses of observational studies of plasma 25-hydroxyvitamin D or 1,25-dihydroxyvitamin D concentrations and **randomized controlled trials of vitamin D supplementation.**

Data sources: Medline, Embase, and screening of citations and references.

Eligibility criteria: Three types of studies were eligible for the umbrella review: systematic reviews and meta-analyses that examined observational associations between circulating vitamin D concentrations and any clinical outcome; and meta-analyses of randomized controlled trials assessing supplementation with vitamin D or active compounds (both established and newer compounds of vitamin D).

Results: 107 systematic literature reviews and 74 meta-analyses of observational studies of plasma vitamin D concentrations and 87 meta-analyses of randomized controlled trials of vitamin D supplementation were identified. The relation between vitamin D and 137 outcomes has been explored, covering a wide range of skeletal, malignant, cardiovascular, autoimmune, infectious, metabolic, and other diseases. Ten outcomes were examined by both meta-analyses of observational studies and meta-analyses of randomized controlled trials, but **the direction of the effect and level of statistical significance was concordant only for birth weight (maternal vitamin D status or supplementation).**

On the basis of the available evidence, **an association between vitamin D concentrations and birth weight, dental caries in children, maternal vitamin D concentrations at term, and parathyroid hormone concentrations in patients with chronic kidney disease requiring dialysis is probable**, but further studies and better designed trials are needed to draw firmer conclusions.

In contrast to previous reports, **evidence does not support the argument that vitamin D only supplementation increases bone mineral density or reduces the risk of fractures or falls in older people.**

Conclusions Despite a few hundred systematic reviews and meta-analyses, **highly convincing evidence of a clear role of vitamin D does not exist for any outcome, but associations with a selection of outcomes are probable.**

Introduction

The associations between vitamin D concentrations and various conditions and diseases have been assessed in a large and rapidly expanding literature. In addition to observational studies, numerous randomized trials have examined the effect of vitamin D supplementation on a range of outcomes.

Historically, vitamin D had been linked to skeletal disease including calcium, phosphorus, and bone metabolism, osteoporosis, fractures, muscle strength, and falls.

In the 2000s, growing scientific attention turned to non-skeletal chronic diseases as vitamin D deficiency was linked to cancer, cardiovascular diseases, metabolic disorders, infectious diseases, and autoimmune diseases, as well as mortality.

If causal, these associations might be of great importance for public health, as vitamin D deficiency has been found to be highly prevalent in populations residing at high latitudes or leading an indoors oriented lifestyle.

However, **the composite literature is often confusing** and has led to heated debates about the optimal concentrations of vitamin D and related guidelines for supplementation.

Methods

Structure of umbrella review

An umbrella review systematically collects and evaluates information from multiple systematic reviews and meta-analyses on all clinical outcomes for which these have been performed. For evidence on randomized controlled trials of vitamin D supplementation, we considered only formal quantitative meta-analyses.

Data extraction

We categorized outcomes into the following categories: autoimmune diseases, cancer outcomes, cardiovascular outcomes, cognitive disorders, infectious diseases, metabolic disorders, neonatal/infant/child related outcomes, pregnancy related outcomes, skeletal outcomes (including falls), and "other" outcomes.

Data analysis

We categorized the conclusions of each systematic review for the association of vitamin D and the outcome of interest in one of the following four categories: **definite association, suggestive (possible) association, no association, or inconclusive (insufficient) evidence.**

Criteria for evidence categories

- *Convincing*—Evidence existed from both observational studies and randomized controlled trials (RCTs), and association/effect was of the same direction, statistically significant at P≤0.001, and free from bias

- *Probable*—Evidence existed from both observational studies and RCTs, and association/effect was of the same direction and statistically significant at P≤0.001, but excess significance could not be tested; or evidence existed from RCTs and effect was statistically significant at P≤0.001 and with no contrary results from observational data

- *Suggestive*—Evidence from RCTs with an effect at 0.001≤ P≤0.05 and with no contrary results from observational data (same as above); *No conclusion*—Not enough evidence from observational studies or RCTs to draw conclusion

- *Substantial effect unlikely*—Evidence from observational studies or RCTs enough to conclude that a substantial effect is unlikely based on the magnitude and the significance level

Results

Overall, 1,256 articles searched yielded 107 systematic reviews without meta-analyses (presented in 24 papers) and 74 meta-analyses (47 papers) of observational studies that investigated associations with circulating vitamin D concentrations. In addition, we identified and included 87 meta-analyses (32 papers) of randomized controlled trials of vitamin D supplementation.

This represents a comprehensive study of the currently available data.

Vitamin D concentrations and health outcomes: systematic reviews of observational studies

For only six (8%) of the 76 unique outcomes, the systematic reviews concluded that a definite association existed. These were rheumatoid arthritis activity, colorectal cancer, hypertension in children, bacterial vaginosis in pregnant women, falls in older people, and rickets in children; for all these outcomes, higher concentrations of vitamin D were associated with lower risk.

Conversely, for 10 (13%) outcomes, the authors concluded that no association existed between the examined outcome and vitamin D status. No systematic reviews concluded that a definite or suggestive association existed for increased risk with higher concentrations of vitamin D.

Meta-analyses of randomized controlled trials of vitamin D supplementation

We identified 87 meta-analyses of randomized controlled trials of vitamin D supplementation. Overall, 13 (23%) of the 57 meta-analyses of randomized controlled trials reported a nominally statistically significant summary result, and these were related to the following outcomes: total cholesterol concentrations, birth weight, head circumference at birth, maternal vitamin D concentrations at term, balance sway, femoral neck bone mineral density, muscle strength, non-vertebral fractures, rate of falls, dental caries in children, parathyroid hormone concentrations in patients with chronic kidney disease (requiring or not requiring dialysis), and risk of hypercalcaemia in patients with chronic kidney disease not requiring dialysis.

Discussion

Our umbrella review identified 107 systematic literature reviews and 74 meta-analyses of observational studies of plasma vitamin D concentrations and 87 meta-analyses of randomized controlled trials of vitamin D supplementation.

The role of vitamin D has been explored in relation to an impressive number of outcomes (137 in total), covering a wide range of diseases, including among others skeletal, malignant, cardiovascular, autoimmune, infectious, and metabolic diseases.

Most of the associations that give signals of nominal significance for diverse outcomes are subject to the caveats that generally accompany evidence from observational studies: many of them may be false positives, and very few, if any, may translate to effective interventions when tested in randomized trials.

On the basis of the results of this umbrella review, **highly convincing evidence of a clear role of vitamin D with highly significant results in both randomized and observational evidence does not exist for any outcome.**

Because of the many misleading advertisements before the public, I repeat the umbrella conclusion for emphasis: on the basis of the results of this umbrella review, **highly convincing evidence of a clear role of vitamin D with highly significant results in both randomized and observational evidence does not exist <u>for any outcome.</u>**

Vitamin D supplementation is <u>probably</u> linked to a decrease in dental caries in children and in parathyroid hormone concentrations in patients with chronic kidney disease requiring dialysis and to an increase in maternal vitamin D concentrations at term and in birth weight.

<u>Suggestive evidence</u> exists for a correlation between high vitamin D concentrations and low risk of colorectal cancer, non-vertebral fractures, cardiovascular disease, prevalence of cardiovascular disease, hypertension, ischemic stroke, stroke, cognition, depression, high body mass index, prevalence of metabolic syndrome, type 2 diabetes, head circumference at birth, small for gestational age birth, and gestational diabetes mellitus; reduced levels of balance sway, alkaline phosphatase concentrations in chronic kidney disease patients requiring dialysis, and parathyroid hormone concentrations in chronic kidney disease patients not requiring dialysis; and increased levels of low density lipoprotein, bone mineral density in femoral neck, and muscle strength.

On the other hand, <u>suggestive evidence exists that high vitamin D concentrations are linked to an increased rate of falls and risk of hypercalcaemia in chronic kidney disease patients not requiring dialysis</u>.

Evidence of relation between high vitamin D concentrations or vitamin D supplementation and clinical outcomes

Most (30/48) of the meta-analyses of observational studies reported a nominally statistically significant result. However, **meta-analyses of**

randomized controlled trials reported a nominally statistically significant summary result for only 13 of the 57 outcomes, and the confidence intervals of the estimates were generally wider than the confidence intervals of the meta-analyses of observational studies.

Genuine differences between these two designs might be due to confounding or biases that operate in observational studies.

Strengths and weaknesses of study and in relation to other studies

As in all literature reviews, the quality is directly related to the quality of the included studies.

Investigators decided to exclude observational meta-analyses of vitamin D supplementation and include only meta-analyses of randomized controlled trials in relation to vitamin D supplementation. **Meta-analyses of randomized controlled trials are subject to considerably less bias than are those of observational studies** and are therefore selected as the standard against which observational meta-analyses of vitamin D concentrations are compared.

Large studies in our review had relatively similar results to other studies and to the summary meta-analysis effect.

As they were preparing their review for submission, a relevant overview of observational studies and randomized controlled trials of vitamin D status or supplementation and ill health was published online. (Autier et al, 2014)

The results of Autier et al, 2014 overview were similar to this umbrella review. Autier's article follows this one.
Possible explanations and implications for clinicians and policy makers

No universal consensus exists on the optimal vitamin D intake or the optimal plasma concentrations of 25-hydroxyvitamin D.

The Institute of Medicine issued a report in 2011 stating that 25-hydroxyvitamin D concentrations of 50 nmol/L are adequate and suggested that these concentrations can be achieved by 600 IU of vitamin D per day. (Ross et al, 2011)

Furthermore, vitamin D supplementation has been long thought to protect against osteoporosis and consequently to reduce the risk and number of fractures, so **large numbers of older adults use vitamin D supplements**. (Bailey et al, 2010)

That nearly half of the meta-analyses of randomized controlled trials were related to skeletal diseases is not surprising. **Several randomized controlled trials have identified a protective effect of vitamin D supplementation (with or without co-administration of calcium) against fractures.** (Bischoff-Ferrari et al, 2005) (Bischoff-Ferrari, et al 2012)

But **trials that examined vitamin D only supplementation <u>failed to replicate</u> these findings**. (Avenell et al, 2009)

Similarly, **a very recent meta-analysis of randomized controlled trials on bone mineral density failed to show a definite association** and **<u>concluded that widespread use of vitamin D supplementation for prevention of osteoporosis is not supported by the evidence</u>, a fact that is also verified by the findings of our review**. (Reid et al, 2014)

Vitamin D might not be as essential as previously thought in maintaining bone mineral density. Similar are our findings for falls, with the results of **two recent Cochrane reviews failing to find a protective effect of vitamin D only supplementation on the risk or rate of falling in older adults** (both in care facilities or hospitals and in the community). (Cameron et al, 2012) (Gillespie et al, 2012)

The lack of convincing associations and the relative dearth of probable associations suggest that evidence for benefits that may be reaped from population-wide vitamin D supplementation is weak.

Probable associations, where highly significant effects appear in randomized trials, hold the most promise for clinical translation, but they pertain to specific populations (children, pregnant women, patients with chronic kidney disease), and **even in these cases the evidence is not sufficient to make universal recommendations about daily intake**. Optimal vitamin D intake/concentration may not be the same for all outcomes.

In addition, **the absorption/metabolism of vitamin D differs among individuals**; in practice, this means that the same supplementation dose is not going to have a stable effect on plasma vitamin D concentration, introducing yet **another source of variability**. Moreover, individual characteristics (such as body mass index or disease) will further modify final concentrations in circulation. In this regard, current recommendations on daily supplementation of vitamin D are largely expert driven, rather than evidence based, and this may be the reason why they have generated so much debate.

Some recommendations that focus on specific outcomes such as prevention of falls and fractures and in which even higher doses of vitamin D are recommended (for example, the American Endocrine Society, Osteoporosis Canada) seem actually to be contradicted by the **evidence, which shows no consistent beneficial effects in randomized trials**.

Our overview of the evidence on vitamin D suggests that strong recommendations cannot be made regarding its supplementation.

Conclusions, unanswered questions, and future research

In conclusion, although vitamin D has been extensively studied in relation to a range of outcomes and some indications exist that low plasma vitamin D concentrations might be linked to several diseases, **firm universal conclusions about its benefits cannot be drawn**.

Randomized controlled trials of vitamin D for autoimmune and cancer related outcomes are clearly lacking.

In addition, earlier evidence from randomized controlled trials that vitamin D supplementation (with or without calcium) increases bone mineral density and reduces the risk of fractures in older people is not seen in clinical trials that examine vitamin D only supplementation.

On the basis of the results of this review, **an association between vitamin D concentrations and birth weight, dental caries in children, maternal vitamin D concentrations at term, and parathyroid hormone concentrations in patients with chronic kidney disease requiring dialysis is probable**, but further studies and better designed trials are needed to draw firmer conclusions.

What is already known on this topic

- The role of vitamin D has been explored both in a large number of observational studies and randomized controlled trials and in relation to a multitude of health outcomes

- The composite literature is often **confusing** and has led to heated debates about the role of vitamin D, the optimal concentrations, and related guidelines for supplementation

Prof Randolph M. Howes MD,PhD

- Recent reports have highlighted the lack of concordance between observational studies and randomized controlled trials, concluding that **vitamin D is more likely to be a correlate marker of overall health and not causally involved in disease**

What this study adds

- This umbrella review collectively presents the evidence from systematic reviews and meta-analyses of observational studies and randomized controlled trials in relation to 137 different outcomes covering a wide range of diseases

- In contrast to previous reports, **the findings cast doubt on the effectiveness of vitamin D only supplementation for prevention of osteoporosis or falls**

- **This review highlights the absence of meta-analyses in relation to autoimmune disease and the absence of meta-analyses of randomized clinical trials of vitamin D supplementation in respect of cancer, cognitive, and infectious disease outcomes**

Vitamin D status and ill health: a systematic review

(Autier et al, 2014)

Summary

Low serum concentrations of 25-hydroxyvitamin D (25[OH]D) have been associated with many non-skeletal disorders. However, **whether low 25(OH)D is the cause or result of ill health is not known.** We did a systematic search of prospective and intervention studies that assessed the effect of 25(OH)D concentrations on non-skeletal health outcomes in individuals aged 18 years or older. We identified 290 prospective cohort studies (279 on disease occurrence or mortality, and 11 on cancer characteristics or survival), and 172 randomized trials of major health outcomes and of physiological parameters related to disease risk or inflammatory status.

Investigators of most <u>prospective studies</u> reported moderate to strong inverse associations between 25(OH)D concentrations and cardiovascular diseases, serum lipid concentrations, inflammation, glucose metabolism disorders, weight gain, infectious diseases, multiple sclerosis, mood disorders, declining cognitive function, impaired physical functioning, and all-cause mortality.

High 25(OH)D concentrations were not associated with a lower risk of cancer, except colorectal cancer.

Results from <u>intervention studies</u> did not show an effect of vitamin D supplementation on disease occurrence, including colorectal cancer.

In 34 intervention studies including 2805 individuals with mean 25(OH)D concentration lower than 50 nmol/L at baseline supplementation with 50 µg per day or more did not show better results. Supplementation in elderly people (mainly women) with 20 µg vitamin D per day **<u>seemed</u>** to slightly reduce all-cause mortality.

The discrepancy between observational and intervention studies **<u>suggests</u> that low 25(OH)D is a marker of ill health.** Inflammatory processes involved in disease occurrence and clinical course would reduce 25(OH)D, which would explain why low vitamin D status is reported in a wide range of disorders. In elderly people, restoration of vitamin D deficits due to ageing and lifestyle changes induced by ill health could explain why low-dose supplementation leads to slight gains in survival.

Effects of vitamin D supplements on bone mineral density: a systematic review and meta-analysis (Reid et al, 2014)

Background

Findings from **recent meta-analyses of vitamin D supplementation without co-administration of calcium have not shown fracture prevention**, possibly because of insufficient power or inappropriate doses, or because the intervention was not targeted to deficient populations. Despite these data, **almost half of older adults (older than 50 years) continue to use these supplements.** We investigated whether vitamin D supplementation affects bone mineral density.

Methods

We searched Web of Science, Embase, and the Cochrane Database, from inception to July 8, 2012, for trials assessing the effects of vitamin D (D3 or D2, but not vitamin D metabolites) on bone mineral density. We included all randomized trials comparing interventions that differed only in vitamin D content, and which included adults (average age >20 years) without other metabolic bone diseases. We pooled data with a random effects meta-analysis with weighted mean differences and 95% CIs reported. To assess heterogeneity in results of individual studies, we used Cochran's Q statistic and the I2 statistic. The primary endpoint was the percentage change in bone mineral density from baseline.

Findings

Of 3,930 citations identified by the search strategy, 23 studies (mean duration 23·5 months, comprising 4082 participants, 92% women, average age 59 years) met the inclusion criteria. 19 studies had mainly white populations. Mean baseline serum 25-hydroxyvitamin D concentration was less than 50 nmol/L in eight studies (n=1791). In ten studies (n=2294), individuals were given vitamin D doses less than 800 IU per day. Bone mineral density was measured at one to five sites (lumbar spine, femoral neck, total hip, trochanter, total body, or forearm) in each study, so 70 tests of statistical significance were done across the studies. **There were six findings of significant benefit, two of significant detriment, and the rest were non-significant.** Only one study showed benefit at more than one site. **Results of our meta-analysis showed a small benefit at the femoral neck with heterogeneity among trials. No effect at any other site was reported, including the total hip.** We recorded a bias toward positive results at the femoral neck and total hip.

Interpretation

Continuing widespread use of vitamin D for osteoporosis prevention in community-dwelling adults without specific risk factors for vitamin D deficiency seems to be inappropriate. (Reid et al, 2014)

Vitamin D not needed for healthy people

Jan 23, 2014

There is little reason to prescribe vitamin D supplements to healthy adults to reduce the risk of diseases or fractures, say researchers writing in the Lancet. **They found no significant reduction in risk in any area after analyzing more than 100 trials.**

They added that future studies were unlikely to change the figures.

At-risk groups, including babies, pregnant women and elderly people, are still advised to take supplements.

The research team, from the **University of Auckland in New Zealand**, had previously carried out a meta-analysis which showed no major effect of vitamin D supplementation on bone mineral density.

"GPs shouldn't be rushing around getting blood tests done for the average healthy person" Quote, Dr Colin Michie Royal College of Pediatrics and Child Health.

In this study, **they looked at existing randomized controlled trials of vitamin D supplements, with or without calcium.**

They found that vitamin D supplementation does not change the relative risk of heart disease, stroke or cerebrovascular disease, cancer and fractures by a noticeable amount, equivalent to 15%.

Vitamin D supplements did not reduce hip fracture risk by more than 15% in hospital patients and, when given with calcium, did not lessen the risk in healthy individuals either.

The study said there was also "uncertainty as to whether vitamin D with or without calcium reduces the risk of death".

The New Zealand researchers concluded: <u>**In view of our findings, there is little justification for prescribing vitamin D supplements to prevent myocardial infarction or ischemic heart disease, stroke or cerebrovascular disease, cancer, or fractures, or to reduce the risk of death in unselected community-dwelling individuals. Investigators and funding bodies should consider**</u>

the probable futility of undertaking similar trials of vitamin D to investigate any of these endpoints. (Bolland et al, 2014)

Far from clear

Writing in a linked article in the Lancet, Karl Michaelsson, from the department of surgical sciences at Uppsala University in Sweden, said there was continuing debate about whether there were health benefits to taking vitamin D supplements for a mild form of vitamin D deficiency.

"The impression that vitamin D is a sunshine vitamin and that increasing doses lead to improved health is far from clear."

Mr Michaelsson said that until more information was available, it would be wise to choose a cautious approach to vitamin D supplementation for otherwise healthy individuals.

While some nutrition experts say vitamin D deficiency is responsible for a number of diseases, such as fractures, cancer, cardiovascular diseases, diabetes, and a higher risk of death, **others say vitamin D deficiency is more likely to be the result of ill health and not the cause**.

Dr Colin Michie, consultant senior lecturer in pediatrics and chairman of the nutrition committee at the Royal College of Pediatrics and Child Health, says the study puts Vitamin D supplements into context.

"This shows vitamin D has a relevant role to play, but it's not that important.

"GPs shouldn't be rushing around getting blood tests done for the average healthy person.

"Instead, the old-fashioned advice still holds true. Eat more fish, watch your diet and how you lead your life - unless you're specifically at risk."

People at high risk of vitamin D deficiency include children under five, pregnant and breastfeeding women, the over-65s and people at risk of not getting enough exposure to sunlight.

Those with darker skin, such as people of African, Caribbean and South Asian origin, and people who wear full-body coverings, as well as pale-skinned people have also been shown to be at higher risk.

Maintain 25(OH)D above 30 nmol/L for bone health of elderly

Hip fractures and bone mineral density in the elderly--importance of serum 25-hydroxyvitamin D

Abstract

BACKGROUND:

The significance of serum 25-hydroxyvitamin D [25(OH)D] concentrations for hip fracture risk of the elderly is still uncertain. Difficulties reaching both frail and healthy elderly people in randomized controlled trials or large cohort studies may in part explain discordant findings. We determined hazard ratios for hip fractures of elderly men and women related to serum 25(OH)D, including both the frail and the healthy segment of the elderly population.

METHODS:

The AGES-Reykjavik Study is a **prospective study of 5,764 men and women**, age 66-96 years, based on a representative sample of the population of Reykjavik, Iceland. Participation was 71.8%. Hazard ratios of incident hip fractures and baseline bone mineral density were determined according to serum concentrations of 25(OH)D at baseline.

RESULTS:

Mean follow-up was 5.4 years. Compared with referent values (50-75 nmol/L), hazard ratios for hip fractures were 2.24 for serum 25(OH)D <30 nmol/L, adjusting for age, sex, body mass index, height, smoking, alcohol intake and season, and 2.08, adjusting additionally for physical activity. **No difference in risk was associated with 30-50 nmol/L or ≥75 nmol/L in either model compared with referent.** Analyzing the sexes separately, hazard ratios were 2.61 in men and 1.93 in women. Values <30 nmol/L were associated with significantly lower bone mineral density of femoral neck compared with referent, z-scores -0.14 in men and -0.11 in women.

CONCLUSIONS:

Our results lend support to the overarching importance of maintaining serum 25(OH)D above 30 nmol/L for bone health

of elderly people while potential benefits of having much higher levels could not be detected. (Steingrimsdottir et al, 2014)

Vitamin D insufficiency in elderly or postmenopausal women

Vitamin D supplementation in elderly or postmenopausal women: a 2013 update of the 2008 recommendations from the European Society for Clinical and Economic Aspects of Osteoporosis and Osteoarthritis (ESCEO).

Abstract

BACKGROUND:

Vitamin D insufficiency has deleterious consequences on health outcomes. In elderly or postmenopausal women, it may exacerbate osteoporosis.

SCOPE:

There is currently no clear consensus on definitions of vitamin D insufficiency or minimal targets for vitamin D concentrations and proposed targets vary with the population. In view of the potential confusion for practitioners on when to treat and what to achieve, the European Society for Clinical and Economic Aspects of Osteoporosis and Osteoarthritis (ESCEO) convened a meeting to provide recommendations for clinical practice, to ensure the optimal management of elderly and postmenopausal women with regard to vitamin D supplementation.

FINDINGS:

Vitamin D has both skeletal and extra-skeletal benefits. Patients with serum 25-hydroxyvitamin D (25-(OH)D) levels <50 nmol/L have increased bone turnover, bone loss, and possibly mineralization defects compared with patients with levels >50 nmol/L. Similar relationships have been reported for frailty, nonvertebral and hip fracture, and all-cause mortality, with poorer outcomes at <50 nmol/L.

CONCLUSION:

The ESCEO recommends that 50 nmol/L (i.e. 20 ng/mL) should be the minimal serum 25-(OH)D concentration at the population level and in patients with osteoporosis to ensure optimal bone health. Below this threshold, supplementation is recommended at 800 to 1000 IU/day. Vitamin D supplementation is safe up to 10,000 IU/day (upper limit of safety) resulting in an upper limit of adequacy of 125 nmol/L 25-(OH)D. Daily consumption of calcium- and vitamin-D-fortified food products (e.g. yoghurt or milk) can help improve vitamin D intake. **Above the threshold of 50 nmol/L, there is no clear evidence for additional benefits of vitamin D supplementation.** On the other hand, **in fragile elderly subjects who are at elevated risk for falls and fracture, the ESCEO recommends a minimal serum 25-(OH)D level of 75 nmol/L** (i.e. 30 ng/mL), for the greatest impact on fracture. (Rizzoli et al, 2013)

This gives an opposing view on the need for vitamin D.

Vitamin D combined with calcium in osteoporosis

Vitamin D and vitamin D analogues for preventing fractures associated with involutional and post-menopausal osteoporosis. (Avenell et al, 2009)

Update in

Cochrane Database Syst Rev. 2014;4:CD000227.

OBJECTIVES:

Investigators tried to determine the effects of vitamin D or related compounds, with or without calcium, for preventing fractures in older people.

SEARCH STRATEGY:

We searched the Cochrane Bone, Joint and Muscle Trauma Group Specialised Register, the Cochrane Central Register of Controlled Trials (The Cochrane Library 2007, Issue 3), MEDLINE, EMBASE, CINAHL, and reference lists of articles. Most recent search: October 2007.

SELECTION CRITERIA:

Randomized or quasi-randomized trials comparing vitamin D or related compounds, alone or with calcium, against placebo, no intervention, or calcium alone, reporting fracture outcomes in older people.

DATA COLLECTION AND ANALYSIS:

Two authors independently assessed trial quality, and extracted data. Data were pooled, where admissible, using the fixed-effect model, or random-effects model if heterogeneity between studies appeared high.

MAIN RESULTS:

Forty-five trials were included. **Vitamin D alone appears unlikely to be effective in preventing hip fracture** (nine trials, 24,749 participants, RR 1.15, 95% CI 0.99 to 1.33), vertebral fracture (five trials, 9138 participants, RR 0.90, 95% CI 0.42 to 1.92) or any new fracture (10 trials, 25,016 participants, RR 1.01, 95% CI 0.93 to 1.09). **Vitamin D with calcium reduces hip fractures** (eight trials, 46,658 participants, RR 0.84, 95% CI 0.73 to 0.96). Although subgroup analysis by residential status showed a significant reduction in hip fractures in people in institutional care, the difference between this and the community-dwelling subgroup was not significant (P = 0.15).

Overall <u>hypercalcaemia is significantly more common in people receiving vitamin D or an analogue, with or without calcium</u>; this is especially true of calcitriol. **There is a modest increase in gastrointestinal symptoms and a small but significant increase in renal disease.**

AUTHORS' CONCLUSIONS:

Frail older people confined to institutions may sustain fewer hip fractures if given vitamin D with calcium.

Vitamin D alone is unlikely to prevent fracture. Overall there is a small but significant increase in gastrointestinal symptoms and renal disease associated with vitamin D or its analogues. Calcitriol is associated with an increased incidence of hypercalcaemia. (Avenell et al, 2009)

Vitamin D dose response in postmenopausal women

Dose response to vitamin D supplementation in postmenopausal women: a randomized trial

Abstract

BACKGROUND:

Serum 25-hydroxyvitamin D (25-[OH]D) is considered the best bio-marker of clinical vitamin D status.

OBJECTIVE:

To determine the effect of increasing oral doses of vitamin D(3) on serum 25-(OH)D and serum parathyroid hormone (PTH) levels in post-menopausal white women with vitamin D insufficiency (defined as a 25-[OH]D level ≤50 nmol/L) in the presence of adequate calcium intake. These results can be used as a guide to estimate the Recommended Dietary Allowance (RDA) (defined as meeting the needs of 97.5% of the population) for vitamin D(3).

DESIGN:

Randomized, placebo-controlled trial. (ClinicalTrials.gov registration number: NCT00472823)

SETTING:

Creighton University Medical Center, Omaha, Nebraska.

PARTICIPANTS:

163 healthy postmenopausal white women with vitamin D insufficiency enrolled in the winter or spring of 2007 to 2008 and followed for 1 year.

INTERVENTION:

Participants were randomly assigned to receive placebo or vitamin D(3), 400, 800, 1600, 2400, 3200, 4000, or 4800 IU once daily. Daily calcium supplements were provided to increase the total daily calcium intake to 1200 to 1400 mg.

MEASUREMENTS:

The primary outcomes were 25-(OH)D and PTH levels at 6 and 12 months.

RESULTS:

The mean baseline 25-(OH)D level was 39 nmol/L. The dose response was curvilinear and tended to plateau at approximately 112 nmol/L in patients receiving more than 3200 IU/d of vitamin D(3). The RDA of vitamin D(3) to achieve a 25-(OH)D level greater than 50 nmol/L was 800 IU/d. A mixed-effects model predicted that 600 IU of vitamin D(3) daily could also meet this goal. Compared with participants with a normal body mass index (<25 kg/m(2)), obese women (≥30 kg/m(2)) had a 25-(OH)D level that was 17.8 nmol/L lower. Parathyroid hormone levels at 12 months decreased with an increasing dose of vitamin D(3) (P = 0.012). Depending on the criteria used, hypercalcemia occurred in 2.8% to 9.0% and hypercalciuria in 12.0% to 33.0% of participants; events were unrelated to dose.

LIMITATION:

Findings may not be generalizable to other age groups or persons with substantial comorbid conditions.

CONCLUSION:

A vitamin D(3) dosage of 800 IU/d increased serum 25-(OH) D levels to greater than 50 nmol/L in 97.5% of women; however, a model predicted the same response with a vitamin D(3) dosage of 600 IU/d. **These results can be used as a guide for the RDA of vitamin D(3)**, but prospective trials are needed to confirm the clinical significance of these results. (Gallagher et al, 2012)

Doubt cast on vitamin D's role against disease

Dec 5, 2013

Vitamin D supplements are recommended for young children and the elderly.

Scientists have cast doubt on the value of vitamin D supplements to protect against diseases such as cancers, diabetes and dementia.

Writing in **The Lancet Diabetes and Endocrinology, <u>French researchers suggest low vitamin D levels do not cause ill health,</u>** although they did not look at bone diseases.

More clinical trials on non-skeletal diseases are needed, they say.

Vitamin D supplements are recommended for certain groups.

Recent evidence has shown it may also have a role to play in preventing non-bone-related diseases such as Parkinson's, dementia, cancers and inflammatory diseases.

Prof Philippe Autier, from the International Prevention Research Institute in Lyon, carried out **a review of data from 290 prospective observational studies and 172 randomized trials looking at the effects of vitamin D levels on health outcomes, excluding bone health, up to December 2012.**

Discrepancy

A large number of the <u>observational studies</u> suggested that there were benefits from high vitamin D - that it could reduce the risk of cardiovascular events by up to 58%, diabetes by up to 38% and colorectal cancer by up to 33%.

But the results of the clinical trials - where participants were given vitamin D supplements - <u>found no reduction in risk</u>, even in people who started out with low vitamin D levels.

And a further analysis of recent randomized trials found no positive effect of vitamin D supplements on diseases occurring.

Prof Autier said: "What this discrepancy suggests is that decreases in vitamin D levels are a marker of deteriorating health."

What is a vitamin D deficiency?

A vitamin D level less than 25nmol/L in the blood is a deficiency, but experts increasingly believe that lower than 60nmol/L can also be damaging to health.

Most people get enough vitamin D by being exposed to the sun for 10 to 15 minutes a day.

Prof Randolph M. Howes MD,PhD

A small amount of vitamin D also comes from foods such as oily fish and dairy products.

Recently England's chief medical officer said free vitamins should be given to all young children because more and more of them were being diagnosed with the bone disease rickets, lack of calcium and other bone and muscle diseases.

"Ageing and inflammatory processes involved in disease occurrence... reduce vitamin D concentrations, which would explain why vitamin D deficiency is reported in a wide range of disorders."

High risk

In the UK, vitamin D supplements are recommended for groups at higher risk of deficiency, including all pregnant and breastfeeding women, children under five years old, people aged over 65, and people at risk of not getting enough exposure to sunlight.

People with dark skin, such as people of African-Caribbean and South Asian origin, and people who wear full-body coverings, as well as pale-skinned people are also known to be at higher risk.

In recent years, there has been a four-fold increase in admissions to UK hospital with rickets - a disease that causes bones to become soft and deformed.

Dr Colin Michie, consultant senior lecturer in pediatrics and chair of the nutrition committee at the Royal College of Pediatrics and Child Health, said the review had little to contribute to the problem in the UK because it excluded the measurement of bone health.

"It has been known for almost a century that vitamin D supplements given to those with deficient vitamin D levels results in improved bone health, preventing hypocalcemic seizure and rickets."

He added that it was important to provide appropriate supplements, such as vitamin D, to improve bone health.

More research

Peter Selby, consultant physician and honorary professor of metabolic bone disease at Manchester Royal Infirmary, said the French review was limited.

"It could very well be that the apparent negative results of this study have been obtained simply because they have not been looking at people with sufficient degree of vitamin D insufficiency to have any meaningful biological effect."

But he said the authors were right to say that more interventional research looking at disease outcomes was necessary.

The Scientific Advisory Committee on Nutrition (SACN), an independent group of scientific experts who advise the government on nutrition, is currently reviewing the dietary recommendations for vitamin D for all population groups in the UK.

Their report on vitamin D is expected to go out for public consultation in 2014.

Vitamins and supplements: save your money

Vitamins and Supplements to Prevent Heart Disease and Cancer? Save Your Money

Henry R. Black, MD April 25, 2014

Dr. Henry Black, Adjunct Professor at the Langone New York University School of Medicine, and a former President of the American Society of Hypertension gave his opinion.

Twenty-eight billion dollars. Does that sound like a lot of money? It does to me. **That is how much Americans spent in 2010 on vitamins and supplements: $28 billion.**

It is very important that we find out whether vitamins and supplements do any good, or whether they do any harm. This is something that the US Preventive Services Task Force (USPSTF) has looked at very carefully. (USPSTF, Moyer et al, 2014) This is an unbiased group that tends to look at the evidence and make recommendations. They are very conservative and very cautious. They looked at vitamin supplements as a package, and at individual vitamins as well, and combinations of a vitamin and a mineral: for example, calcium and vitamin D.

It's no surprise to me that they found that **almost none of them did what that was promised.** This includes vitamin C, which was thought to prevent heart attacks and cancer, not to mention colds. It includes vitamin E, which was supposed to prevent almost everything. **Every time this has been looked at, there was no evidence that these supplements worked**. Beta-carotene, for example, which was supposed to prevent cancer and heart disease, turned out probably to be harmful, especially for lung cancer in high-risk groups.

Why do we do buy and take supplements? It makes some sense biologically. In some small studies and in some animal studies, they acted as antioxidants, which would be very useful to prevent heart disease and cancer. But when you actually put them to the test in humans -- the only experimental animal that really matters, in my opinion -- you just don't see those results. I don't think these were malicious attempts to sell to people things that they didn't need, but **when we look at the evidence, vitamins and supplements don't necessarily work.**

Individual vitamins have been looked at, and some have benefits. For example, folic acid in women who are pregnant seems to prevent neural tube disorders. Vitamin D in older individuals, especially women, seems to be particularly helpful. Much of that evidence comes from the **Women's Health Initiative, where we had a large number of older women and there was a reduction in fractures in the women who took vitamin D**. (Jackson et. al, 2006) (Prentice et al, 2013

Whether vitamin D needs to be taken with calcium remains to be seen.

The problem is that we don't test these things the way that we test everything else. The multivitamin preparations are wildly different -- different doses, different anions, different cations -- so it's very hard to sort this out. **Right now, there is a belief system that supplements are good. It's hard to challenge that belief system** without evidence that they aren't good, but we have to consider this very carefully.

I have been told that doctors don't recommend vitamins. Doctors who tend to be evidence-based aren't going to recommend something that they don't feel have proof that it works.

There are harms too that we should know about, such as the fact that **calcium and vitamin D tend to increase calcium stones.** That is something that we found in the Women's Health Initiative as well, and it was not surprising. That fits with what we knew about how those compounds work.

Right now, we have to be very cautious when we are recommending or not recommending vitamins. Inform our patients and our families that the data on using these aren't there right now. Maybe someday they will be; maybe not. **The USPSTF just updated recommendations that they had made in 2003. If anything, they are more strongly certain that beta-carotene is harmful and that there is no evidence of other supplements being helpful.**

Be careful. If you go down to GNC (or other supplement stores), keep your hands on your wallet. Thank you very much.

Healthy adults do not need to take vitamin D supplements, suggests a study in The Lancet which **found they had no beneficial effect on bone density, a sign of osteoporosis**.

But experts say many other factors could be at play and people should not stop taking supplements.

University of Auckland researchers **analyzed 23 studies involving more than 4,000 healthy people.**

The UK government recommends children and over-65s take a daily supplement.

The New Zealand research team conducted a meta-analysis of all randomized trials examining the effects of vitamin D supplementation on bone mineral density in healthy adults up to July 2012.

The supplements were taken for **an average of two years** by the study participants.

"I'm not surprised they didn't find any evidence of the effects of vitamin D on bone density because there are so many other factors involved..." Quote Dr Laura Tripkovic University of Surrey.

Bone mineral density is a measure of bone strength and measures the amount of bone mineral present at different sites in the body. It is often seen as an indicator for the risk of osteoporosis, which can lead to an increased risk of fracture.

The trials took place in a number of different countries including the UK, the US, Australia, Holland, Finland and Norway.

Although the results did not identify any benefits for people who took vitamin D, **they did find a small but statistically significant**

increase in bone density at the neck of the femur near the hip joint.

According to the authors, this effect is unlikely to be clinically significant.

Free up resources

Prof Ian Reid, lead study author, from the University of Auckland, said the findings showed that **healthy adults did not need to take vitamin D supplements**.

"Our data suggest that the targeting of low-dose vitamin D supplements only to individuals who are likely to be deficient could free up substantial resources that could be better used elsewhere in healthcare."

Writing about the study in The Lancet, Clifford J Rosen from the Maine Medical Research Institute agrees that science's understanding of vitamin D supports the findings for healthy adults, but not for everyone.

"Supplementation to prevent osteoporosis in healthy adults is not warranted. However, maintenance of vitamin D stores in the elderly combined with sufficient dietary calcium intake remains an effective approach for prevention of hip fractures."

The Department of Health currently recommends that a daily supplement of vitamin D of 10 micrograms (0.01mg) should be taken by pregnant and breastfeeding women and people over 65, while babies aged six months to five years should take vitamin drops containing 7 to 8.5 micrograms (0.007-0.0085mg) per day.

Additional factors

Dr Laura Tripkovic, research fellow in the department of nutritional sciences at the University of Surrey, said the study was important but very specific.

"I'm not surprised they didn't find any evidence of the effects of vitamin D on bone density because there are so many other factors involved in osteoporosis, like genes, diet and environment."

"To pin it all on vitamin D... it's difficult to do that."

Dr Tripkovic said it was no good taking vitamin D supplements if people didn't also maintain a healthy, balanced diet containing calcium and take plenty of exercise.

She said most healthy people should be able to absorb enough vitamin D naturally, through sunshine and diet.

"But if people are worried about their vitamin D levels then a multi-vitamin tablet would do. If you have bone pain and muscle aches then you should go and see your GP and discuss it."

We get most of our vitamin D from sunlight on our skin, but it is also found in certain foods like oily fish, eggs and breakfast cereals.

However, **taking too much vitamin D in the form of supplements can be harmful because calcium can build up and damage the kidneys**.

Experts advise taking no more than 25 micrograms (0.025mg) a day.

The UK guidance is currently being reviewed.

SECTION THREE

POSITIVE STUDIES: SCIENCE BASED EVIDENCE

'D' Levels Linked to Cancer Death Risk Only in Survivors

Neil Osterweil

June 20, 2014

People with low vitamin D levels are at increased risk of dying from cancer — but only if they have already had cancer, report the authors of a meta-analysis.

All-cause mortality was 1.57 times higher among older adults in the lowest quintile of 25-hydroxyvitamin D [25(OH)D] level, but cancer-related deaths were significantly higher only among persons in that grouping with a history of cancer.

The study also showed, however, that **levels of 25(OH)D are all over the map, varying considerably by country, sex, and time of year**, note Ben Schöttker, PhD, from the Division of Clinical Epidemiology and Aging Research at the German Cancer Research Center in Heidelberg, and colleagues.

"Results from a long term randomized controlled trial addressing longevity are being awaited before vitamin D supplementation can be recommended in most individuals with low 25(OH)D levels," they write in a *BMJ* **open-access** study published online.

In an interview with *Medscape Medical News*, coauthor Paolo Boffetta, MD, MPH, director of the Institute for Translational Epidemiology and professor of hematology and medical oncology at Mount Sinai Hospital in New York City, said that the investigators are not sure why they saw an effect of vitamin D only in patients with a history of cancer.

"One specific aspect of our study was that it was conducted in the elderly population, so we had a large proportion of people with a previous cancer," which could have skewed results, Dr. Boffetta said.

"Whether vitamin D may be particularly related to risk of multiple cancers or some general susceptibility to cancer which may be related to reaction to inflammatory conditions, this is the sort of thing we speculated about. But this is the first time that this has been reported, and clearly it needs to be confirmed in other investigations, particularly in elderly cohorts," he said.

The *BMJ* editors note that the study hints at a role of vitamin D in cancer prognosis and suggests that for clinical purposes, cutoff values for determining vitamin D deficiency many need to be customized by geography, age, sex, and season.

However, a cancer specialist is not so sure about the prognostic value of vitamin D.

"I agree that the study might be interpreted 'from either side' as supporting a role for vitamin D deficiency in cancer risk — though only in prior cancer patients — or it can be viewed as demonstrating lack of correlation or weakness of correlation overall," commented David E. Fisher, MD, PhD, Edward Wigglesworth Professor and chairman of the Department of Dermatology, Harvard Medical School, and director of the Melanoma Program at Massachusetts General Hospital Cancer Center in Boston.

He was not involved in the study and was asked for comment.

"As pointed out by the authors, a 'reverse' correlation cannot be ruled out (i.e., multicancer patients may be more prone to become vitamin D deficient). I believe the studies, while somewhat provocative, do not support an obvious role for vitamin D in cancer prevention," Dr. Fisher said.

D and Death: A Mixed Picture

As reported by *Medscape Medical News*, another recent meta-analysis of 17,000 cancer patients in China found better overall survival for patients with lymphoma, colorectal cancer, or breast cancer who were in the highest quartile of circulating 25(OH)D levels compared with lowest quartile.

Higher circulating levels of vitamin D were also significantly associated with lower cancer-specific mortality rates among patients with both colorectal cancer and lymphoma, and disease-free survival rates were also significantly improved for patients with breast cancer and those with lymphoma.

A different meta-analysis, also recently reported, found that women with high levels of vitamin D in their blood when they were diagnosed with breast cancer were almost twice as likely to survive as those with low levels of vitamin D.

But **vitamin D skeptics can point to yet another meta-analysis looking at vitamin D supplements for the prevention of myocardial infarction, stroke, cancer, or hip fracture in seniors, which found that, in general, taking vitamin D does not lower the incidence of these outcomes.**

In the current study, the investigators consolidated data on 26,018 participants from the age of 50 to 79 years in 7 European **cohorts and one US study (the National Health and Nutrition Examination Survey III).**

Mean follow-up times in the studies ranged from 4.2 to 15.9 years. During follow-up, 6695 participants died — 2227 from cancer, 2624 from cardiovascular diseases, and the remainder from other causes.

To account for variations in vitamin D levels across the regions and cohorts in the study, the investigators defined 25(OH)D quintiles with cohort- and subgroup-specific cutoff values.

They found that all-cause mortality in the lowest vs highest quintiles was 1.5 times higher.

But **when they looked at cancer-specific mortality, they found a significant association only for those with a history of cancer.**

There was a consistent inverse dose-response trend seen across the studies for all-cause and cardiovascular mortality and for cancer mortality in patients with a history of cancer.

Prof Randolph M. Howes MD,PhD

D Still Gets Good Grade

Although the relationship between vitamin D and mortality may be fuzzy, the benefits for D in overall health are clear, Dr. Fisher emphasized.

"From a dermatology perspective, I would add that vitamin D is solidly established to be important for other medical/health reasons, especially pertaining to calcium and bone metabolism. Therefore, establishing and maintaining a healthy vitamin D level is part of good health maintenance," he told *Medscape Medical News*.

"I would add that this should be done by measuring blood levels of vitamin D and if necessary using oral supplements to achieve the necessary levels. Sun exposure as a means of establishing a healthy vitamin D level is both dangerous (carcinogenic) and unreliable (due to variations in sun intensity, skin pigmentation, geographical location, time of day, etc)," he wrote.

The meta-analysis was part of the CHANCES project, funded by a grant from the European Commission. The authors and Dr. Fisher reported no relevant financial relationships.

BMJ. 2014;348:g3656.

Study links low vitamin D levels with premature death

Friday 13 June 2014

In recent months, there has been much debate surrounding vitamin D. Some studies have suggested that a high level of the vitamin benefits our health, while others have reported that there is not enough evidence to make such a claim. Now, a new study from the University of California-San Diego School of Medicine suggests a link between vitamin D deficiency and early death.

Vitamin D is a fat-soluble **vitamin** that helps regulate the absorption of **calcium** and phosphorus in our bones, as well as aid cell communication and strengthen the immune system.

Researchers have long associated vitamin D deficiency with poor bone health. In fact, three years ago, the US Institute of Medicine (IOM) concluded that **low vitamin D is hazardous because it signifi-cantly increases the risk of bone disease.**

But the health problems associated with vitamin D deficiency do not stop there. Last year, *Medical News Today* reported on a study led by the University of Kentucky, which indicated that **vitamin D deficiency may damage the brain.** More recent research claimed that low levels of vitamin D in the first 26 weeks of pregnancy **may increase the risk of preeclampsia.**

For this latest study, published in the *American Journal of Public Health*, the UC-San Diego team wanted to see how vitamin D deficiency influenced mortality rates.

Subjects with lower vitamin D levels 'twice as likely to die prematurely'

The researchers conducted a systemic review of 32 studies that analyzed vitamin D, blood levels and mortality rates. The studies involved 566,583 participants from 14 counties - including the US - who were an average age of 55.

Participants' 25-hydroxyvitamin D levels were assessed. This is the main form of vitamin D found in human blood.

Results of the study revealed that participants with lower levels of 25-hydroxyvitamin D in their blood were twice as likely to die prematurely, compared with those who had higher blood levels of 25-hydroxyvitamin D. (Garland et al, 2014)

Furthermore, the team found that the 25-hydroxyvitamin D blood level associated with approximately half of participants who were at higher risk of early death was 30 ng/ml - a level that around two thirds of Americans are already below.

According to the National Institutes of Health, children and adults ages 1-70 should have 600 IU (international units) of vitamin D each day, while adults over this age should have 400 IU a day.

But according to study co-author Heather Hofflich, professor in the Department of Medicine at the UC-San Diego School of Medicine:

"This study should give the medical community and public substantial reassurance that vitamin D is safe when used in appropriate doses up to 4,000 IU per day," says study co-author Heather Hofflich.

However, she adds that patients should have their 25-hydroxyvitamin D blood levels checked annually and consult their doctor before adjusting their vitamin D intake.

Not all researchers are so positive about increasing vitamin D intake. Earlier this year, *Medical News Today* reported on two studies published in the *BMJ*, which suggested that there is **"no clear evidence"** that **vitamin D benefits health**.

Another study, published in *The Lancet Diabetes & Endocrinology* in January, also **questioned the health benefits of vitamin D**, after an assessment of 40 randomized controlled trials revealed that vitamin D supplements are unlikely to reduce the incidence of **heart attack, heart disease, stroke, cancer** and **bone fractures**.

Study author Dr. Mark Bolland, of the University of Auckland in New Zealand, commented:

"The main message is that if you are otherwise healthy and active, you are likely to receive enough sunshine to have adequate vitamin D levels and don't need to take vitamin D supplements."

Written by Honor Whiteman http://www.medicalnewstoday.com/articles/278120.php Accessed 6-13-14.

The study was conducted by researchers from the University of California, San Diego School of Medicine. They analyzed 32 studies that were previously conducted on vitamin D, blood levels and human mortality rates. All the studies looked at a specific variant of vitamin D called 25-hydroxyvitamin D, the primary form found in blood.

"Three years ago, the Institute of Medicine (IOM) concluded that having a too-low blood level of vitamin D was hazardous," said Cedric Garland, DrPH, lead author of the study in a press statement. "This study supports that conclusion, but goes one step further. The 20 nanograms per milliliter (ng/ml) blood level cutoff assumed from the IOM report was based solely on the association of low vitamin D with risk of bone disease. This new finding is based on the association of low vitamin D with risk of premature death from all causes, not just bone diseases."

Researcher noted that **the vitamin D level in the blood associated with premature deaths was 30 ng/ml.** What's concerning is that **two-thirds of the U.S. population has an estimated blood vitamin D level below 30 ng/ml.**

Though many recent studies have highlighted the negative consequences of excessive vitamin D in the blood, the findings of this study suggest that the nutrient is safe when used in appropriate doses up to 4,000 International Units (IU) per day. Study authors recommend getting 25-hydroxyvitamin D levels checked annually. Also, anyone making changes in their Vitamin D consumption should first seek advice from their doctors.

Many of the previously touted benefits of vitamin D have been questioned lately. A study conducted in March this year noted that the vitamin is not effective in reducing depression risks, debunking previous beliefs.

Another study found no concrete evidence to suggest that vitamin D supplements are effective in preventing accidental falls in older people.

In January this year, University of Auckland researchers released a controversial report suggesting healthy people may not benefit as much from Vitamin D as it doesn't have a significant effect on preventing heart attacks, stroke, cancer or bone fractures in such people.

In another report, **the U.S. National Cancer Institute noted that its studies conducted on the effects of vitamin D on cancer may not be completely accurate because studying a person's blood vitamin level at a single point in time, as many studies do, may not give an accurate picture of his or her true levels. Moreover, many studies don't use high enough doses to see the benefits.**

Despite this, various studies and health experts continue to vouch for the health benefits of vitamin D and how it can help in keeping serious health issues at bay. **Very recently, Northwestern University researchers said that vitamin D can help reduce the risk of aggressive prostate cancer in men.**

The current study was funded by the UC San Diego Department of Family and Preventive Medicine. Findings were published online in the American Journal of Public Health.

Prof Randolph M. Howes MD,PhD

Regulation of T cell by vitamin D

Regulation of T cell development and function by vitamin D

Autoimmune diseases like multiple sclerosis (MS) and inflammatory bowel disease (IBD) occur because of an inappropriate immune-mediated attack against self-tissue. Analyses of genetically identical twins shows that besides genetics there are important environmental factors that contribute to MS and IBD development. Vitamin D availability due to sunshine exposure or diet may play a role in the development of MS and IBD. Compelling data in mice show that vitamin D and signaling through the vitamin D receptor dictate the outcome of experimental MS and IBD. Furthermore, **the evidence points to the direct and indirect regulation of T cell development and function by vitamin D.** In the absence of vitamin D and signals delivered through the vitamin D receptor, auto reactive T cells develop and in the presence of active vitamin D (1,25(OH)(2)D(3)) and a functional vitamin D receptor the balance in the T cell response is restored and autoimmunity avoided. (Cantorna, 2006)

Immune system is under the influence of vitamin D

Abstract

Multiple sclerosis (MS) is a chronic demyelinating disease and also is one of the most common disabling neurological disorders in young and middle-aged adults. The main pathogenesis of MS has long been thought to be an immune mediated disorder of the central nervous system. **The function of the immune system is under the influence of vitamin D which as a modulator of immune response could play a role in autoimmune diseases including MS.** Deficiency of vitamin D or variations in DNA sequence (polymorphism) of vitamin D receptor gene diminishes its optimal function on immune system that consequently could lead to increasing risk of MS. However, its role in development and modulating the course of MS is still under investigation. In this review we aimed to discuss the role of vitamin D in body, immune system and consequently altering the risk of MS. (Harandi et al, 2014)

Vitamin D and multiple sclerosis

(Harandi et al, 2014) (

Vitamin D is a potent modulator of immune system therefore vitamin D deficiency is the most prominent candidate for MS and is focus of interest in field of MS during recent years.

Vitamin D as an immune modulator

Vitamin D is a steroid hormone that has multiple regulatory and functional effects throughout the body. Vitamin D endocrine system has a central role in control of bone and calcium homeostasis. It can be obtained either through dietary intake and supplements or produced endogenously. It found in foods such as oily fish, egg yolks, fortified milk and juice.

However dietary intake accounts only for about 30% of the vitamin D obtained and is not biologically active, therefore **the main route for obtaining vitamin D is exposure to ultraviolet B sunlight at wavelengths between 290–315 nm** that occur predominantly in the summer months.

The biologically active form of vitamin D is 1,25-dihydroxyvitamin D3 (1,25(OH)2D3) that is produced in several steps. The most of vitamin D is obtained by skin in a UVB-induced process in which 7-dehydrocholesterol convert to vitamin D3 followed by two hydroxylations.

First, in the liver, and then in the kidneys by 25 and 1 hydroxylases, respectively. Finally active metabolite can enter the cell, bind to the vitamin D-receptor and subsequently to a responsive gene.

A central role of 1,25(OH)2D3 is modulation of immune response. This is suggested by the fact that many immune cells including monocytes, macrophages, dendritic cells and activated T and B cells contain vitamin D receptors. It control infections by promoting differentiation of monocytes to macrophages, and enhance their chemotactic and phagocytotic capacity and antibacterial activity.

It also has a preventive role against autoimmunity by reducing the expression of major histocompatibility complex (MHC) class II and co-stimulatory receptors on antigen presenting cells. It acts as a co-stimulatory molecules on monocytes and T cells. Furthermore, 1,25-(OH)2D3 induces proliferation of B cells, differentiation of plasma cells, secretion of immunoglobulin E and M, production of memory B cells, and apoptosis in activated B cells.

In addition it promotes T regulatory cells and reduces T cell proliferation, inhibits production of pro-inflammatory cytokines. Overall, **existing data indicate that 1,25-(OH)2D3 modulates several players of the immune cascade to generate a more anti-inflammatory and tolerogenic profile.**

It has been cleared that treatment by 1,25(OH)2D3 suppress the development of Th1-mediated autoimmune diseases. In addition, treatment of mice with MS symptoms by 1,25(OH)2D3, interrupt the development of the disease in these mice.

Such findings may explain that vitamin D can change the immune response even after the disease had been established.

T cells and ultimately B cells, both may be subject as a direct or indirect targets of 1,25-(OH)2D3. Increasing of vitamin D receptor expression after T cell activation support this hypothesis that T cells are main targets of 1,25-(OH)2D3. However, different activation stimuli appear to evoke diverse vitamin D receptor (VDR) expression levels and kinetics, which may explain the inconsistency in data concerning the effects of 1,25-(OH)2D3 on T cell proliferation.

In addition, 1,25(OH)2D up-regulate many genes such as osteocalcin, osteopontin, calbindin, and 24-hydroxylase. For example, vitamin D metabolites may also have a protective role against diabetes mellitus type 1 by down-regulation of dendritic and Th1 cells, suppression of the antigen-presenting capacity of macrophages and dendritic cells and promotion of Th2 lymphocytes.

More recent findings have also linked vitamin D deficiency to a range of non-skeletal conditions such as cardiovascular disease, cancer, stroke, cognitive impairment and dementia. 1,25(OH)2D has shown neuroprotective effects including the clearance of amyloid plaques, a hallmark of Alzheimer's Disease.

An association has been noted between low 25-hydroxyvitamin D [25(OH)D] and Alzheimer's disease and dementia in both Europe and the United States.

Vitamin D and auto-immune disease

The role of vitamin D has been investigated in several autoimmune diseases, including inflammatory bowel disease (IBD), autoimmune thyroiditis, rheumatoid arthritis (RA), type I diabetes mellitus, mixed connective tissue disease, scleroderma, systemic lupus erythematosus (SLE), allergic encephalomyelitis and MS. It prevents development of autoimmune diseases in animal models. Some studies suggest that risk of some disease such as rheumatoid arthritis, and diabetes mellitus type I, reduce in human with high vitamin D intake.

The best indicator of vitamin D status, reflecting intake from all sources, is serum 1,25-(OH)2D3. Serum levels of less than 25 nmol/L considered as severely deficient, levels between 25-80 nmol/L considered as insufficient of mildly to moderately deficient and levels more than 80 nmol/L considered as sufficient.

Patients with MS have low serum levels of vitamin D compared to the international norm, and it has been hypothesized vitamin D plays an immune-modulatory role in the CNS, perhaps through a Th1-mediated response.

Vitamin D deficiency not linked to early thyroid autoimmunity

Abstract

CONTEXT:

Vitamin D deficiency has been identified as a risk factor for a number of autoimmune diseases including type I diabetes and multiple sclerosis.

OBJECTIVE:

We hypothesized that low levels of vitamin D are related to the early stages of autoimmune thyroid disease (AITD).

DESIGN:

Two case-control studies were performed. In the cross-sectional study A, euthyroid subjects with genetic susceptibility for AITD but without thyroid antibodies were compared with controls. Cases were subjects from the Amsterdam AITD cohort (euthyroid women who had first- or second-degree relatives with overt AITD) who at baseline had normal TSH and no thyroid antibodies; controls were healthy women examined at the same period. In the longitudinal study B, subjects who developed de novo thyroid peroxidase antibody (TPO-Ab) were compared with those who did not. Cases and controls were subjects from the Amsterdam AITD cohort who at baseline had normal TSH and no thyroid antibodies and during follow-up developed TPO-Ab (cases) or remained without thyroid antibodies (controls). Controls in both studies were matched for age, BMI, smoking status, estrogen use, month of blood sampling, and in study B for the duration of follow-up.

RESULTS:

Serum 25(OH)D levels were as follows: study A: 21.0 ± 7.9 vs 18.0 ± 6.4 ng/ml; study B: baseline, 22.6 ± 10.3 vs 23.4 ± 9.1; follow-up 21.6 ± 9.2 vs 21.2 ± 9.3 ng/ml.

CONCLUSIONS:

Early stages of thyroid autoimmunity (in study A genetic susceptibility and in study B development of TPO-Ab) are not associated with low vitamin D levels. (Effraimidis et al, 2012)

Vitamin D is an in vitro potent immune modulator, that can ameliorate, or even cure, animal models with MS. (Note: this is questionable.)

In the other word, a poor vitamin D status could increase risk for MS and lead to a more severe disease course of MS. Several experimental studies, have shown that vitamin D brings the immune system in a less pro-inflammatory state. This important role of vitamin D in preventing immune deviation has been argued to underlie the association of a poor vitamin D status with MS. However, the causality of this association is not thoroughly clear.

Risk factors for vitamin D deficiency

The most common risk factors for vitamin D deficiency are low sun exposure, skin pigmentation, premature and dysmature birth, obesity, malabsorption, race, age and environmental factors.

Vitamin D deficiency is much more frequent in Europe than in Asia and America. In Europe, the highest serum 25(OH)D3 levels were observed in Scandinavian countries and the lowest levels were found in Mediterranean countries that may be due to high sun exposure, a light skin and multivitamin use in northern countries while shadow-seeking behavior and a darker skin are more common in Mediterranean countries.

A high prevalence of vitamin D insufficiency has been reported in Afro-Americans, because people with dark-colored skin have a reduced ability to synthesize vitamin D upon exposure to sunlight than those with light-colored skin.

Also prevalence of vitamin D deficiency is high in non-western immigrants in the Netherlands and in the Middle East especially in Iran, where life-style factors probably play a role.

Because of changes that occur with aging, older people with any other risk factors for vitamin D deficiency are likely to have inadequate stores of this vitamin. Elderly individuals also have a lower capacity to synthesize vitamin D on exposure to ultraviolet-B radiation and often stay indoors.

People hospitalized for a long time and are not supplemented with vitamin D and people who wear concealing clothing for religious or cultural purposes may be at higher risk of vitamin D deficiency. Supplementation with cod-liver oil had a protective role in person with low summer outdoor activities.

Vitamin D2 is not a suitable supplement for many reasons including absorption, differences in efficacy at raising vitamin D levels, diminished binding to proteins in blood, shorter shelf-life etc.

Vitamin D deficiency is common in patients with MS.

Some recent research studies suggest that a lack of vitamin D in early childhood or before birth might increase the risk of developing MS (multiple sclerosis) later in life. Outdoor activities during summer in early life (ages 16–20 years) were associated with a decreased risk of MS. Epidemiological study showed that women with the highest supplements of vitamin D intakes had a 40% reduction in the risk of developing MS comparing women with intake of >400 IU/day to those with no supplemental vitamin D. A dose of 1000 to 4000 IUs daily to achieve a serum level of > 99nmol/L is safe and may reduce MS risk by as much as 62% MS.

Prof Randolph M. Howes MD,PhD

Conclusion

The maintenance of adequate vitamin D levels has important influence on different aspects of health and well- being. Vitamin D deficiency is a modifiable risk factor for MS and because of its role in control of immune responses almost certainly has some beneficial effects on disease course in MS. Several studies revealed prominent role of Vitamin D in immune mediated diseases like MS. (Harandi et al, 2014)

Vitamin D has unknown effect on thyroid diseases

Elevated anti-thyroid antibodies had lower levels of serum 25(OH)D3

Abstract

PURPOSE:

The association between autoimmune thyroid diseases (AITDs) and vitamin D deficiency is controversial. We aimed to evaluate the relationship between serum 25-hydroxy-vitamin D3 [25(OH)D3] and anti-thyroid antibody levels.

MATERIALS AND METHODS:

25(OH)D3, anti-thyroid antibodies, and thyroid function measured in 304 patients who visited the endocrinology clinic were analyzed. The patients were subgrouped into the AITDs or non-AITDs category according to the presence or absence of anti-thyroid antibodies. The relationship between anti-thyroid peroxidase antibody (TPOAb) and 25(OH)D3 was evaluated.

RESULTS:

The patients with elevated anti-thyroid antibodies had lower levels of serum 25(OH)D3 than those who did not. Importantly, after adjusting for age, sex, and body mass index, a negative correlation was recognized between 25(OH)D3 and TPOAb levels in the AITDs group, but this correlation did not exist in the non-AITDs group. 25(OH)D3 level was confirmed as an independent factor after adjusting for co-factors that may affect the presence of TPOAb in the AITDs group.

CONCLUSION:

25(OH)D3 level is an independent factor affecting the presence of TPOAb in AITDs. The causal effect of 25(OH)D3 deficiency to AITDs is to be elucidated. (Shin et al, 2014)

Low vitamin D in pre-menopausal women with AITD

Vitamin D deficiency related to pre-menopausal women with autoimmune thyroid disease (AITD)

Abstract

BACKGROUND:

Low serum vitamin D levels have been associated with several autoimmune diseases, but their association with thyroid autoimmunity is unclear. We evaluated the association of serum vitamin D levels with the prevalence of autoimmune thyroid disease (AITD).

METHODS:

Our cross-sectional study included subjects who underwent routine health checkups, which included assays of serum 25-hydroxy vitamin D3 [25(OH)D3] and anti-thyroid peroxidase antibody (TPO-Ab), as well as thyroid ultrasonography (US) between 2008 and 2012 at the Asan Medical Center. We defined AITD according to the levels of TPO-Ab and US findings.

RESULTS:

A total of 6685 subjects (58% male; 42% female) were enrolled for this study. Overall prevalence of TPO-Ab positivity and both TPO-Ab/US positivity were 10.1% and 5.4% respectively. In female subjects, mean serum 25(OH)D3 levels were significantly lower in the TPO-Ab(+) and TPO-Ab(+)/US(+) groups compared with the control group, respectively. According to the levels of serum 25(OH)D3, the prevalence of TPO-Ab positivity and both TPO-Ab and US positivity decreased in female subjects. Interestingly, **this pattern was significant only in pre-menopausal women (p=0.003 and p<0.001; respectively), but not in postmenopausal women.** Multivariate analysis indicated that the adjusted odds ratios (OR) for AITD among those in the 25(OH)D3-deficient and -insufficient groups were significantly increased when compared with the sufficient group.

CONCLUSIONS:

The levels of serum vitamin D were significantly lower in pre-menopausal women with AITD. Vitamin D deficiency and insufficiency were significantly associated with AITD in pre-menopausal women. Low levels of serum vitamin D3 are associated with autoimmune thyroid disease in pre-menopausal women. (Choi et al, 2014)

Vitamin D's early role with TB

Sunlight and vitamin D played an early role in preventing and treating TB.

In the early 20th century, TB patients were often sent to sanatoria in the mountains where they were exposed to solar radiation. Dr. Auguste Rollier set up such facilities in the Swiss Alps. (Hobday, 1997)

Sun exposure is associated with a lower incidence of TB six months later. (Koh et al, 2012)

It wasn't until 2006-7 that researchers at UCLA determined how sunlight increased vitamin D levels and helps the body's immune system prevent bacterial infections. (Liu et al, 2007)

Higher blood levels of 25-hydroxyvitamin D can reduce the time required to control TB during treatment. (Coussens et al, 2012)

Recent research suggests the sanatoria approach to treatment could have been at least partly effective.

TB and Vitamin C

Despite the data strongly suggesting the impact of nutrition, corporate medicine has consistently decried the use of supplements. Recently, however, there has been a long overdue development. Catherine Vilchèze and colleagues have returned to testing the extraordinary antibiotic properties of vitamin C for TB.

They was found that "M. tuberculosis is highly susceptible to killing by vitamin C" which is consistent with previous data. Notably, **the mechanism of action is similar to vitamin C's anticancer role in generating hydrogen peroxide locally which kills the unwanted cells.** Notably, we have been using antibiotic treatment of TB as a model for the role of vitamin C based redox therapy for cancer. **The same mechanism is used to protect the body against both microorganisms and abnormal cancer cells.** (Hickey, Roberts, 2013)

Supplementation with vitamin C may prevent TB infection from becoming overt. Furthermore, vitamin C could provide an effective biological treatment for TB with the advantage of a mechanism refined by millions of years of evolution. As scientific history demonstrates, good nutrition, particularly vitamins C and D, are likely to be far more effective than antibiotics and vaccination in preventing this and other dangerous infective diseases.

Vitamin D reduces cancer risk - 2011 study

Studies on breast and colorectal cancer found that an increase of serum 25(OH)D concentration of 10 ng/ml was associated with a 15% reduction in colorectal cancer incidence and 11% reduction in breast cancer incidence. (Gandini et al, 2011) http://www.ncbi.nlm.nih.gov/pubmed/20473927. **Yet, this has been basically debunked by newer RCTs. I included this study to show the conflicted results.**

Vitamin D increases breast cancer survival - 2012 study

Women diagnosed with breast cancer had increased survival for those with higher serum 25(OH)D concentrations. In those with lower vitamin D concentrations, mortality increased by 8%. (Vrieling et al, 2012) http://www.ncbi.nlm.nih.gov/pubmed/21791049.

Andrew W. Saul's Timeline of vitamin medicine

1951 - Vitamin D treatment is found to be effective against Hodgkin's disease (a cancer of the lymphatic system) and epithelioma.

1963 - Vitamin D is shown to prevent breast cancer.

1964 - Vitamin D is found to be effective against lymph nodal reticulo-sarcoma (a non-Hodgkin's lymphatic cancer).

2011 - Each 20 micromole/liter (µmol/L) increase in plasma vitamin C is associated with a 9% reduction in death from heart failure. Also, B complex vitamins are associated with a 7 percent decrease in mortality, vitamin D with an 8 percent decrease in mortality.

Orthomolecular Medicine News Service, February 15, 2014.

However, many of these assertions have been currently questioned due to additional scientific studies.

Vitamins 'effective in treating ADHD symptoms'

1-30-14 Could micronutrients such as zinc, calcium and vitamins improve brain functioning?

Vitamins and minerals could be useful for treating ADHD, **research suggests**.

Adults with ADHD given supplements for eight weeks had a "modest" improvement in concentration span, hyperactivity, and other symptoms, a small-scale study found.

A wide range of nutrients, including vitamin D, iron and calcium, **may** improve brain functioning, said psychologists in New Zealand.

Another study found medication reduced road accidents in men with ADHD.

As many as one in 20 adults has ADHD (attention-deficit hyperactivity disorder), marked by symptoms such as lack of attention, concentration difficulties and impulsiveness.

ADHD can be treated with medications, such as central nervous system stimulants, which affect the brain and improve symptoms.

"The risk of transport accidents in adult men with ADHD decreases markedly if their condition is treated with medication" Quote, Prof Henrik Larsson, Karolinska Institute.

According to the research, published in **The British Journal of Psychiatry, taking a broad range of vitamins and minerals may also help reduce ADHD symptoms.**

In the study, 80 adults with ADHD were given either supplements containing vitamin D, vitamin B12, folate, magnesium, ferritin, iron, calcium, zinc and copper, or a dummy pill. (Published in JAMA Psychiatry.)

After eight weeks of treatment those on supplements reported greater improvements in both their inattention and hyperactivity/impulsivity compared with those taking the placebo.

Psychologists from the University of Canterbury, in Christchurch, say **the effects of vitamins and minerals (micronutrients) are more modest than medication but may be useful for some people, particularly those seeking alternative treatments.**

"Our study provides preliminary evidence of the effectiveness for micronutrients in the treatment of ADHD symptoms in adults," said Prof Julia Rucklidge, who led the study.

"This could open up treatment options for people with ADHD who may not tolerate medications, or do not respond to first-line treatments."

Philip Asherson, professor in molecular psychiatry at the Institute of Psychiatry in London, said **the suggestion that vitamins and minerals improved brain metabolism was intriguing but needed further investigation.**

Prof Randolph M. Howes MD,PhD

"It's a good study, which is very interesting, but really needs replicating," he told the BBC. "The mechanisms behind it remain unclear."

A similar effect was not found in women.

"Even though many people with ADHD are doing well, our results indicate that the disorder may have very serious consequences," said Henrik Larsson, associate professor at the Department of Medical Epidemiology and Biostatistics.

"Our study also demonstrates in several different ways that the risk of transport accidents in adult men with ADHD decreases markedly if their condition is treated with medication."

Adults with ADHD given supplements for eight weeks had a "modest" improvement in concentration span, hyperactivity, and other symptoms, a small-scale study found.

A wide range of nutrients, including vitamin D, iron and calcium, may improve brain functioning, said psychologists in New Zealand.

Vitamin D increases breast cancer patient survival - 2014 discussion

3/7/2014

Breast cancer patients with high levels of vitamin D in their blood are twice as likely to survive the disease as women with low levels of this nutrient, report University of California, San Diego School of Medicine researchers in the March issue of Anticancer Research. Garland and colleagues performed a statistical analysis of five studies of 25–hydroxy-vitamin D obtained at the time of patient diagnosis and their follow–up for an average of nine years.

Combined, the studies included 4,443 breast cancer patients. "Vitamin D metabolites increase communication between cells by switching on a protein that blocks aggressive cell division," said Garland. "As long as vitamin D receptors are present tumor growth is prevented and kept from expanding its blood supply. Vitamin D receptors are not lost until

124

a tumor is very advanced. This is the reason for better survival in patients whose vitamin D blood levels are high."

Vitamin D may raise cancer survival rates

Among breast, colorectal and other cancers, Vitamin D may raise survival rates

May 1, 2014

Cancer patients who have higher levels of vitamin D when they are diagnosed tend to have better survival rates and remain in remission longer than patients who are vigtamin D-deficient, according to a new study published in the Endocrine Society's *Journal of Clinical Endocrinology & Metabolism (JCEM)*.

The body naturally produces vitamin D after exposure to sunlight and absorbs it from certain foods. In addition to helping the body absorb the calcium and phosphorus needed for healthy bones, vitamin D affects a variety of biological processes by binding to a protein called a vitamin D receptor. This receptor is present in nearly every cell in the body.

"By reviewing studies that collectively examined vitamin D levels in 17,332 cancer patients, our analysis demonstrated that vitamin D levels are linked to better outcomes in several types of cancer," said one of the study's authors, Hui Wang, MD, PhD, Professor of the Institute for Nutritional Sciences at the Shanghai Institutes for Biological Sciences at the Chinese Academy of Sciences in Shanghai, China. **"The results suggest vitamin D may influence the prognosis for people with breast cancer, colorectal cancer and lyphoma, in particular."**

The meta-analysis looked at the results of **25 separate studies** that measured vitamin D levels in cancer patients at the time of diagnosis and tracked survival rates. In most of the research, patients had their vitamin D levels tested before they underwent any treatment for cancer. **The study found a 10 nmol/L increase in vitamin D levels was tied to a 4 percent increase in survival among people with cancer.**

Researchers found the strongest link between vitamin D levels and survival in breast cancer, lymphoma and colorectal cancer.

There was less evidence of a connection in people with lung cancer, gastric cancer, prostate cancer, leukemia, melanoma or Merkel cell carcinoma, but the available data were positive.

"Considering that **vitamin D deficiency is a widespread issue all over the world**, it is important to ensure that everyone has sufficient levels of this important nutrient," Wang said. "Physicians need to pay close attention to vitamin D levels in people who have been diagnosed with cancer."

Vitamin D is a steroid vitamin, a group of fat-soluble prohormones, which encourages the absorption and metabolism of calcium and phosphorus.

Vitamin D deficiency may predict aggressive prostate cancer

5-1-14

Past research has associated low levels of vitamin D with a number of health problems. Now, a new 2014 study published in the journal *Clinical Cancer Research* suggests that vitamin D deficiency may be an indicator of aggressive prostate cancer.

According to study author Dr. Adam B. Murphy, assistant professor in the Department of Urology at the Northwestern University Feinburg School of Medicine in Chicago, IL, **vitamin D is known to impact the growth and differentiation of benign and malignant prostate cells, both in prostate cell lines and animal models of prostate cancer.**

However, their study revealed that **low levels of the vitamin in men appeared to predict the risk of aggressive prostate cancer.**

To reach their findings, the team enrolled **275 European-American men and 273 African-American men** to the study between 2009 and 2013.

The men were aged between 40 and 79 years and were undergoing an initial prostate biopsy after abnormal prostate-specific antigen (PSA) or digital rectal examination (DRE) test results. A prostate cancer diagnosis from their biopsy was given to 168 men from each group.

In order to determine the levels of vitamin D in the men, the researchers measured levels of **25-hydroxyvitamin D (25-OH D)** in their blood. **The normal range of 25-OH D is 30 to 80 nanograms per milliliter (ng/ml).**

The lower the vitamin D levels, the higher the risk of aggressive prostate cancer.

Researchers found an association between low vitamin D levels and increased risk of aggressive prostate cancer, particularly for African-American men.

The team found that **the mean 25-OH D levels of African-American men were much lower than that of European-American men,** at 16.7 ng/ml and 19.3 ng/ml, respectively.

The highest 25-OH D level found in European-American men was 71 ng/ml, while the highest level found in African-American men was only 45 ng/ml.

The researchers then divided the men into groups dependent on their 25-OH D levels. They were:

- Less than 12 ng/ml

- Less than 16 ng/ml

- Less than 20 ng/ml

- Less than 30 ng/ml.

They found that the lower a man's vitamin D levels, the higher their risk of prostate cancer.

With 25-OH D levels lower than 12 ng/ml, European-American men were 3.66 times more likely to develop aggressive prostate cancer (Gleason grade 4+4 or higher), while African-American men were 4.89 times more likely to develop an aggressive form of the disease.

European-American men were also 2.42 times more likely to have a stage T2b tumor (when cancer can be felt or seen on scans but is contained within the prostate) if 25-OH D were less than 12 ng/ml, while African-American men were 4.22 times more likely to have a stage T2b tumor.

Prof Randolph M. Howes MD,PhD

Furthermore, **the researchers found that African-American men were also 2.43 times more likely to be diagnosed with prostate cancer if their 25-OH D levels were less than 20 ng/ml**. No association was found between vitamin D deficiency and increased risk of prostate cancer diagnosis in European-American men.

A person's main source of vitamin D is from the sun, and skin color can affect how much is absorbed. The researchers say this may explain why African-American men appear to have increased risk of prostate cancer diagnosis and an aggressive form of the disease.

Speaking of the next steps for this research, Dr. Murphy says:

It seems men's health really is affected by low levels of vitamin D.

Another study recently reported by *Medical News Today* suggests that **low vitamin D levels may be associated with chronic widespread pain in men.**

Written by Honor Whiteman http://www.medicalnewstoday.com/articles/276190.php?tw

The following was taken from a 2014 Vitamin D continuing medical education release:

Note: some of the material in this CME release are not in agreement with recent RCTs but I will let it stand or fall on its own merits.

High vitamin D improves breast cancer survival - CME

High Vitamin D Levels Yield Improved Breast Cancer Survival - CME

News Author: Fran Lowry

CME Author: Laurie Barclay, MD

CME Released: 03/31/2014

Dr. Mohr, Dr. Garland, and Dr. Murphy

Clinical Context

Among women worldwide, breast cancer is the most prevalent cancer, with 1.7 million new cases and approximately half a million deaths in 2012. Previous research has examined the association between vitamin D levels and breast cancer incidence.

However, the association between serum 25-hydroxyvitamin D (25[OH]D) status and breast cancer survival rates remains unclear. The objective of this meta-analysis by Mohr and colleagues was to pool findings from previous studies of this association.

Study Synopsis and Perspective

Women with high levels of vitamin D in their blood when they are diagnosed with breast cancer are almost twice as likely to survive as those with low levels of vitamin D, according to a meta-analysis published in the March issue of *Anticancer Research*.

The meta-analysis looked at 5 studies of serum 25(OH)D levels that reported hazard ratios for mortality from breast cancer by quintiles of the vitamin. Combined, the studies involved 4,443 patients with breast cancer.

For an average of 10 years, breast cancer mortality rate was 44% lower in patients in the quintile with the highest levels of serum 25(OH)D than in the quintile with the lowest levels.

For the 5 studies, the pooled hazard ratio summarizing the estimated risk for breast cancer mortality in the lowest quintile, compared with the highest quintile, was 0.56 ($P < .0001$).

In 3 of the studies, fatality rates were substantially lower in the highest quintile than in the lowest quintile. In 2 of the studies, there was a trend in that direction.

"Doctors should emphasize the importance of maintaining adequate serum vitamin D levels, which would be 40 to 60 ng/mL for cancer prevention, and encourage their patients to have their vitamin D status regularly checked, especially in winter, to ensure that adequate serum levels are being maintained," said first author Sharif B. Mohr, MD, from the Naval Health Research Center in San Diego, California.

For women already diagnosed with breast cancer, vitamin D levels could go as high as 80 ng/mL, he told *Medscape Medical News*.

Prof Randolph M. Howes MD,PhD

Studies have already established that vitamin D prevents breast and colon cancer, "so every adult should ensure that they maintain adequate serum levels of vitamin D, either through moderate sun exposure or by taking vitamin D₃ supplements," he said.

A previous study of Canadian women with breast cancer found that those who had very low levels of vitamin D when they were diagnosed were more likely to have aggressive disease, as previously reported by *Medscape Medical News*. In fact, women with very low levels of vitamin D at diagnosis were 94% more likely to have metastases than women with normal levels, and 73% were more likely to die.

Vitamin D Stops Tumor Growth

"Vitamin D makes cells stick together, particularly breast epithelial cells, by producing upregulation of the synthesis of E-cadherin," senior author Cedric F. Garland, DrPH, from the Department of Family and Preventive Medicine at the University of California, San Diego, told *Medscape Medical News*.

"If the vitamin D level gets low, the cells of the breast epithelium don't adhere to each other, and when a cell is not tightly adherent to its neighbors, its stem cells undergo rapid mitosis," Dr. Garland explained. "The cells that reproduce the fastest can produce a cancerous clone, which can ultimately penetrate the basal membrane. If the vitamin D deficiency continues, those cells will get out into the lymphatics, metastasize to the brain, bone, and lungs, and kill the patient."

However, "with a lot of vitamin D, the cells are self-adherent and never evolve into a cancer," he noted. "If it's late in the history and they have evolved into a cancer, it will be a well-differentiated cancer. Those are not as aggressive as the poorly differentiated cells that will eventually break through a blood vessel and kill people. As long as the cells have a vitamin D receptor intact — and most cells do because it's a very robust receptor — the vitamin D will make the tumor stop growing. It will freeze it in its track," he said.

Doctors should measure vitamin D levels in their breast cancer patients. If the levels are deficient, these patients should immediately be given 40,000 IU of vitamin D daily to get it up to 40 to 60 ng/mL, Dr. Garland advised.

It is also crucial to measure serum calcium levels, which should be 8.5 to 10.2 mg/dL, he said.

"A woman should receive 1500 mg of calcium along with her vitamin D, because there are clinical trials showing that vitamin D works best when accompanied by that dose of calcium. Calcium is best if it is taken from food, although it's very hard to get it out of vegetables," Dr. Garland said.

Finally, he recommended randomized controlled clinical trials to confirm the findings of this meta-analysis. "Numerous studies on the safety of vitamin D_3 are available that would make such a strategy worth considering," he said.

Deficiency Linked to Aggressive Prostate Cancer

"This study is interesting," said Adam B. Murphy, MD, MPH, from the Northwestern University Feinberg School of Medicine in Chicago, Illinois, who was not involved with the meta-analysis.

"Our lab recently showed that **vitamin D deficiency is linked to aggressive features on prostate cancer biopsy**," he told *Medscape Medical News.*

"This study suggests that vitamin D is associated with mortality from breast cancer on meta-analysis," Dr. Murphy noted. "Given the associations with aggressive disease in breast cancer and prostate cancer, this is biologically plausible."

He mentioned that reverse causation "could be at play." This point is also made by Dr. Garland and colleagues, who note that clinical trials are needed to confirm that the association they found between reduced breast cancer mortality and high vitamin D levels is not the result of reverse causation.

Recently, **a large review of clinical trials concluded that low vitamin D levels are the result of various health disorders, not the cause of the health disorders.**

A prospective study of patients with newly diagnosed breast cancer or a randomized clinical trial of vitamin D supplementation that measures rates of recurrence and mortality could be the next step, Dr. Murphy added.

Dr. Mohr, Dr. Garland, and Dr. Murphy have disclosed no relevant financial relationships.

Anticancer Res. 2014;34:1163-1166. Abstract

Study Highlights

- This meta-analysis included 5 studies of the association between 25(OH)D levels and breast cancer mortality.

- These studies enrolled a total of 4443 patients with breast cancer.

- A random-effects model allowed calculation of a pooled hazard ratio, and homogeneity was evaluated with use of the Der Simonian-Laird test.

- Higher serum concentrations of 25(OH)D were associated with lower case-fatality rates after breast cancer diagnosis.

- During follow-up (mean duration, 10 years), mortality rate from breast cancer in the highest quintile of 25(OH)D levels was approximately half (44% lower) than that in the lowest quintile.

- The pooled hazard ratio for estimated breast cancer mortality risk in the lowest vs the highest quintile of 25(OH)D levels was 0.56 (P < .0001).

- 3 of the 5 studies showed significantly lower fatality rates in the highest vs the lowest quintile, whereas 2 of the studies showed a nonsignificant trend favoring lower fatality rates in the highest vs the lowest quintile.

- A limitation of this study is possible reverse causation, if serum 25(OH)D concentration is reduced in more serious cases of breast cancer with early mortality, and if serum 25(OH)D is therefore a biomarker for cancer severity.

- On the basis of their findings, the investigators concluded that high serum levels of 25(OH)D were associated with lower mortality rates from breast cancer. However, they recommend clinical or field studies to confirm that this association was not the result of reverse causation.

- The authors also recommend that all patients with breast cancer undergo restoration of serum 25(OH)D levels to the normal range (30 - 80 ng/mL), with appropriate monitoring.

- The investigators suggest that mechanisms by which vitamin D metabolites may prevent breast cancer may also explain better survival duration in patients with breast cancer who have higher serum 25(OH)D levels when diagnosed.

- Tumor growth might be arrested at almost any point in its cycle from initiation to metastasis by restoration of a high serum 25(OH) D concentration, resulting in upregulation of E-cadherin and restoration of a well-differentiated state.

Clinical Implications

- According to a meta-analysis of 5 previous studies, high serum 25(OH)D levels were associated with lower mortality rates from breast cancer.

- The investigators recommend that serum 25(OH)D levels in all patients with breast cancer be restored to the normal range, with appropriate monitoring.

Red grapes, blueberries and vitamin D may enhance immunity

Immune function likely enhanced by red grapes, blueberries (enhanced by vitamin D)

Sept 19, 2013

In an analysis of 446 compounds for their ability to boost the innate immune system in humans, researchers in the Linus Pauling Institute at Oregon State University discovered **just two that stood out from the crowd - the resveratrol found in red grapes and a compound called pterostilbene from blueberries**.

Both of these compounds, which are called stilbenoids, worked in synergy with vitamin D and had a significant impact in raising the expression of the human cathelicidin antimicrobial peptide, or CAMP gene, that is involved in immune function.

The findings were made in laboratory cell cultures and do not prove that similar results would occur as a result of dietary intake, the scientists said, but do add more interest to the potential of some foods to improve the immune response.

The research was published in *Molecular Nutrition and Food Research*, in studies supported by the National Institutes of Health.

"Out of a study of hundreds of compounds, **just these two popped right out**," said Adrian Gombart, an LPI principal investigator and associate professor in the OSU College of Science. "Their synergy with vitamin D to increase CAMP gene expression was significant and intriguing. It's a pretty interesting interaction."

Resveratrol has been the subject of dozens of studies for a range of possible benefits, from improving cardiovascular health to fighting cancer and reducing inflammation. This research is the first to show a clear synergy with vitamin D that increased CAMP expression by several times, scientists said.

The CAMP gene itself is also the subject of much study, as it has been shown to play a key role in the "innate" immune system, or the body's first line of defense and ability to combat bacterial infection. The innate immune response is especially important as many antibiotics increasingly lose their effectiveness.

A strong link has been established between adequate vitamin D levels and the function of the CAMP gene, and the new research suggests that certain other compounds may play a role as well.

Stilbenoids are compounds produced by plants to fight infections, and in human biology appear to affect some of the signaling pathways that allow vitamin D to do its job, researchers said. **It appears that combining these compounds with vitamin D has considerably more biological impact than any of them would separately**.

Continued research could lead to a better understanding of how diet and nutrition affect immune function, and possibly lead to the development of therapeutically useful natural compounds that could boost the innate immune response, the researchers said in their report.

Despite the interest in compounds such as resveratrol and pterostilbene, their bioavailability remains a question, the researchers said. Some applications that may evolve could be with topical use to improve barrier defense in wounds or infections, they said.

The regulation of the CAMP gene by vitamin D was discovered by Gombart, and researchers are still learning more about how it and other compounds affect immune function. **The unique biological pathways involved are found in only two groups of animals - humans and non-human primates.** Their importance in the immune response could be one reason those pathways have survived through millions of years of separate evolution of these species. (Vit D, blueberries, 2013)

Vitamin D may enhance vaccines

Vitamin D would actually make vaccines work better

Allegedly, you can beat the minimal protective benefits of vaccines with a simple, low-cost vitamin D supplement. Vitamin D, you see, is the nutrient that activates your immune system to fight off infectious disease. Without it, vaccines hardly work at all.

In fact, the very low rate of vaccine efficacy (1%) is almost certainly due to the fact that most people receiving the vaccines are vitamin D deficient. (some say anywhere from 75% - 95% of Americans are deficient in vitamin D, depending on whom you ask.)

Hilariously, the way to make vaccines work better would be to hand out vitamin D supplements to go along with the shots! **Even more hilariously, if people were taking vitamin D supplements, they wouldn't need the vaccine shots in the first place!**

Influenza vaccines, in other words, have no important role whatsoever in preventing influenza infections. **This goal can be accomplished more safely, reliably and at far lower cost by promoting vitamin D supplements for the population at large.**

What we really need to see from the scientific world is a study comparing vitamin D supplements to influenza vaccines **(and using realistic vitamin D doses, not just 200 or 400 IUs per day). Some have absolutely no doubt that healthy-dose vitamin D supplementation (4000 IUs a day) would prove to be significantly more effective than influenza vaccines at preventing flu infections.**

But such a study will almost certainly never be done (at least not anytime soon) because it would expose the false propaganda of the vaccine industry while giving consumers a far better way of protecting themselves from influenza that doesn't involve paying money to vaccine manufacturers.

In medicine, as in war, truth is often the first casualty. And when the lies are repeated with enough frequency, they begin to be believed. The flu shot lie has been repeated with such ferocity and apparent authority that it has snookered in virtually the entire "scientific" community.

Strong associations of 25-hydroxyvitamin D concentrations with all-cause, cardiovascular, cancer, and respiratory disease mortality in a large cohort study.

Schöttker B, Haug U, Schomburg L, Köhrle J, Perna L, Müller H, Holleczek B, Brenner H. Conclusion: In this large cohort study, serum 25(OH)D concentrations were inversely associated with all-cause and cause-specific mortality. In particular, vitamin D deficiency [25(OH)D concentration <30 nmol/L] was strongly associated with mortality from all causes, cardiovascular diseases, cancer, and respiratory diseases.

Vitamin D may reduce CVD mortality

Relationship between 25-hydroxyvitamin D and all-cause and cardiovascular disease mortality.

Amer M, Qayyum R.

Conclusion: We found an inverse association between 25(OH)D and all-cause and cardiovascular disease mortality in healthy adults with serum 25(OH)D levels of ≤21 ng/mL. Clinical trials for the primary prevention of cardiovascular disease with 25(OH)D supplementation may target healthy adults with serum 25(OH)D levels of ≤21 ng/mL to validate these findings.

25-Hydroxyvitamin D Levels and the Risk of Mortality in the General Population

Michal L. Melamed, MD, MHS; Erin D. Michos, MD, MHS; Wendy Post, MD, MS; Brad Astor, PhD. Conclusion: The lowest quartile of 25(OH)D level (<17.8 ng/mL) is independently associated with all-cause mortality in the general population.

Mercola recommends vitamin D for osteoarthritis

February 07, 2014

By Dr. Mercola Vitamin D: Cartilage loss in your knees, **one of the hallmarks of osteoarthritis, is associated with low levels of vitamin D.** So if you're struggling with joint pain due to osteoarthritis, get your vitamin D level tested, then optimize it using appropriate sun exposure or a safe tanning bed. If neither of these options is available, you may want to consider oral vitamin D3 and K2 supplements.

Sun exposure is your best option, because your skin produces two types of sulfur in response to sun exposure: cholesterol sulfate and vitamin D3 sulfate. Sulfur plays a vital role in the structure and biological activity of both proteins and enzymes. If you don't have sufficient sulfur in your body, this deficiency can create a number of health problems, including negative impacts on your joints and connective tissue. Which brings us to the next item...

Please remember that Dr. Mercola aggressively sells dietary supplements.

NICE recommends optimum vitamin D levels

The National Institute for Health and Clinical Excellence (NICE) recommends certain supplements for some groups of people who are at risk of deficiency, including:

• **Folic acid for all women thinking of having a baby and pregnant women up to week 12 of the pregnancy.**

• **Vitamin D for all pregnant and breastfeeding women, children aged six months to five years, people aged 65 and over**

and for people who are not exposed to much sun, for example people who cover up their skin for cultural reasons, or people who are housebound for long periods of time.

• Finally a supplement containing vitamins A, C and D is recommended for all children aged six months to four years. This is a precaution because growing children may not get enough, especially those not eating a varied diet, such as fussy eaters.

• **Optimize your vitamin D levels.** Vitamin D influences virtually every cell in your body and is one of nature's most potent cancer fighters. Vitamin D is actually able to enter cancer cells and trigger apoptosis (cell death). If you have cancer, your vitamin D level should probably be between 70 and 100 ng/ml. Vitamin D works synergistically with every cancer treatment I'm aware of, with no adverse effects.

• Ideally, your levels should reach this point by exposure to the sun or a safe tanning bed, not oral vitamin D. (Note: this is a controversial statement)

SECTION FOUR

GENERAL DISCUSSION

I have summarized the positive and negative studies on vitamin D as follows:

POSITIVE SUPPORT DATA

- A 25(OH)D level of less than 32 ng/mL is considered vitamin D insufficient.

- A 25(OH)D level of less than 20 ng/mL has been used to define vitamin D deficiency.

The way doctors measure if you're deficient in vitamin D is by testing your 25(OH)D level, but most doctors just call this a vitamin D test. Getting this blood test is the only accurate way to know if you're deficient or not. (Holick, 2010) (Plum et al, 2010)

- Vitamin D2 is ergocalciferol

- Vitamin D3, 25(OH)D is cholecalciferol

- Calcitriol is 1,25-dihydroxyvitamin D

- Serum 25(OH)D (1 ng/mL = 2,5 nmol/L) is the barometer for the medical laboratory evaluation of the vitamin D status. 25-hydroxyvitamin D [25(OH)D] is also known as calcidiol.

- The metabolically active vitamin D hormone is [1α,25(OH)$_2$D].

- 1α,25(OH)$_2$D is like the sex hormones (e.g., estradiol) and corticosteroids (e.g., cortisone), which are all steroid hormones.

- The serum 25(OH)D level should be between 30 and 100 ng/mL.

- A 25(OH)D status between 40 and 60 ng/mL or 100 to 150 nmol/L is ideal.

- A pronounced vitamin D deficiency is present at 25(OH)D levels below 20 ng/mL, with levels between 21–29 ng/mL designated as moderate vitamin D deficiency, also referred to as vitamin D insufficiency.

- With a UV index of less than 3, no vitamin D synthesis can take place in the skin.

- Vitamin D intake in the diet plays only a minor role in the vitamin D supply.

- Approximately 1 billion people worldwide are affected by a vitamin D deficiency. [25-OH-D: <20 ng/mL] or a vitamin D insufficiency [25(OH)D: 21–29 ng/mL].

(Grober et al, 2013)

According to the Institute of Medicine (IOM), the current recommended dietary intake of 600 IU for adults under the age of 70 years and 800 IU for adults over 70 years is sufficient to meet the needs of 97.5% of healthy adults who have minimal sun exposure.

The IOM defines sufficiency of 25(OH)D as greater than 20 ng/mL. The IOM, however, noted a concern for attaining levels above 50 ng/mL and designated 4,000 IU daily as the tolerable upper intake limit.

The normal range of 25-OH D is 30 to 80 nanograms per milliliter (ng/ml).

The Vitamin D Council recommends a much higher daily intake of 5,000 IU to achieve a sufficiency level of 50 ng/mL.

The Institute of Medicine issued a report in 2011 stating that 25-hydroxyvitamin D concentrations of 50 nmol/L are adequate and suggested that these concentrations can be achieved by **600 IU of vitamin D per day**. (Ross et al, 2011)

A 2005 Cochrane review found unclear evidence that vitamin D alone affected hip, vertebral, or other fracture rates but supported the use of vitamin D with calcium in frail, elderly nursing home residents. (Avenell et al, 2005) A subsequent 2007 meta-analysis of trials looking at vitamin D and fracture rates concurred that calcium was also necessary to affect a significant difference. (Bonnen et al, 2007)

Several randomized controlled trials have identified a protective effect of vitamin D supplementation (with or without co-administration of calcium) against fractures. (Bischoff-Ferrari et al, 2005) But **trials that examined vitamin D only supplementation <u>failed to replicate</u> these findings.** (Avenell et al, 2009)

Retrospective trials show that vitamin D supplementation is associated with decreased mortality in people on dialysis. (Wolf et al, 2007) However, there have been no randomized prospective trials examining this relationship as of 2007. (Al-Aly, 2007)

Low serum vitamin D levels are also related to increased mortality in most patients with chronic kidney disease before dialysis. (Inaquma et al, 2008)

In patients not on dialysis, low vitamin D levels are associated with increased levels of inflammation and oxidative load. A prospective study of more than 3,000 male and female patients found a positive association between low vitamin D levels and cardiovascular as well as all-cause mortality. (Dobnig et al, 2008)

A 2007 meta-analysis demonstrated that intake of a vitamin D supplement at normal doses also was associated with decreased all-cause mortality rates. (Autier, Gandini, 2007) But, causality has not been determined.

During a period of 5 years, participants from the Framingham offspring study who had **25-OH D levels of <15 were more likely to experience cardiovascular events.** The relationship remained significant among people with hypertension but not among those without hypertension. (Wang et al, 2008)

One meta-analysis showed a relatively consistent association between low vitamin D status, calcium or dairy intake, and

prevalence of type 2 DM or metabolic syndrome. (Pittas et al, 2007)

A 2008 evidence summary found that vitamin D supplementation at doses of more than 700 IU daily (plus calcium) prevented bone loss. (Cranney et al, 2008)

A 2004 review of 12 randomized, controlled trials studying the effect of vitamin D supplementation on fall risk among both nursing home residents and community dwellers found a small benefit of supplementation on fall risk. (Bischoff_Ferrari et al, 2004). A 2008 randomized, controlled trial from Australia evaluated women with at least one fall in the preceding 12 months and with a plasma 25-hyroxyvitamin D level <24.0 ng/mL. (Prince et al, 2008) **Women in the study group** (calcium 1000 mg per day) **had fewer falls after 12 months, but this was not a significant difference. Lower doses of vitamin D, however, did not significantly change the rate of fall incidence compared with placebo.** (Broe et al, 2007)

Observational studies in 2008 showed that **people with Alzheimer dementia have lower vitamin D levels than do matched controls without dementia.** (Buell et al, 2008). **A cross-sectional study of 225 outpatients diagnosed with Alzheimer disease found a correlation between vitamin D levels (but not other vitamin levels) and their score on a Mini Mental Status Examination.** (Oudshoom et al, 2008)

The recent 2009 meta-analysis of 12 randomized, controlled trials that included more than 42,000 people found that vitamin D supplementation of more than 400 IU daily slightly reduced incidence of nonvertebral fractures. (Bischoff-Ferrari et al, 2009) The effect was dose dependent and was not significant if doses were ≤400 IU daily.

A Norwegian case-control study found that **fish and cod liver oil have a protective effect against the development of MS**. A large observational study in the United States that followed 2 large cohorts of women—the Nurses' Health Study (92,253 women followed from 1980 to 2000) and the Nurses' Health Study II (95,310 women followed from 1991 to 2001)—found that **vitamin D supplementation in the form of a multivitamin seemed to lower their MS risk by 40%.** (Munger et al, 2004) However, several methodological weaknesses in study design made the results inconclusive. (Smolders et al, 2008)

A 2009 case-control study compared the serum vitamin D levels of 103 multiple sclerosis (MS) patients with 110 controls and found that **for every 10-nmol/L increase of serum 25(OH)D level the odds of MS was reduced by 19% in women, suggesting a "protective" effect of higher vitamin D levels.** (Kragt et al, 2009)

As for chronic pain studies, in those that blinded the vitamin D therapy, only 10% of patients were in trials showing a benefit of vitamin D treatment, whereas among those who did not blind the treatment, 93% were in trials showing a benefit of vitamin D supplementation. (Straube et al, 2009). A second review found **a direct correlation between vitamin D deficiency and musculoskeletal pain.** Treatment of vitamin D deficiency produced an increase in muscle strength and a marked decrease in back and lower-limb pain within 6 months. But, **the available evidence does not imply causality.**

Vitamin D supplementation is <u>probably</u> linked to a decrease in dental caries in children and in parathyroid hormone concentrations in patients with chronic kidney disease requiring dialysis and to an increase in maternal vitamin D concentrations at term and in birth weight. (Vitamin D, Umbrella review, 2014)

<u>Suggestive evidence</u> exists for a correlation between high vitamin D concentrations and low risk of colorectal cancer, non-vertebral fractures, cardiovascular disease, prevalence of cardiovascular disease, hypertension, ischemic stroke, stroke, cognition, depression, high body mass index, prevalence of metabolic syndrome, type 2 diabetes, head circumference at birth, small for gestational age birth, and gestational diabetes mellitus; reduced levels of balance sway, alkaline phosphatase concentrations in chronic kidney disease patients requiring dialysis, and parathyroid hormone concentrations in chronic kidney disease patients not requiring dialysis; and increased levels of low density lipoprotein, bone mineral density in femoral neck, and muscle strength. (Vitamin D, Umbrella review, 2014)

In children, vitamin D deficiency can result in rickets, and there is evidence to show that this condition is re-emerging in the UK. (Lowdon, 2011)

Low circulating levels of the vitamin were associated with increased risk of death from cardiovascular disease, cancer, and other causes, and that supplementation with vitamin D3 cut

mortality risk by 11% (but supplementation with vitamin D2 did not). (Chowdhury et al, 2014)

Participants with lower levels of 25-hydroxyvitamin D in their blood were twice as likely to die prematurely, compared with those who had higher blood levels of 25-hydroxyvitamin D. (Garland et al, 2014) **The vitamin D level in the blood associated with premature deaths was 30 ng/ml.** What's concerning is that two-thirds of the U.S. population has an estimated blood vitamin D level below 30 ng/ml.

Higher blood levels of 25-hydroxyvitamin D can reduce the time required to control TB during treatment. (Coussens et al, 2012)

CANCER (positive studies)

In the 2006 Health Professionals Follow-Up study (a cohort study of 1095 men), each increment in 25(OH)D level of 25mmol/L was associated with a 17% reduction of total cancer cases. (Giovannucci et al, 2006)

However, the National Health and Nutrition Examination Survey of 16,818 men and women did not find a relationship between total cancer mortality and vitamin D level. There was an inverse relationship between vitamin D level and colorectal cancer, however. In this study, serum 25(OH)D levels of ≥80 nmol/L conferred a 72% reduction in risk of colorectal cancer compared with a level lower than 50 nmol/L. (Freedman et al, 2007)

A 2006 meta-analysis of 63 observational studies looked at the relationship between vitamin D levels and cancer incidence and mortality. **Twenty of the 30 studies looking at vitamin D and colon cancer showed that people with higher vitamin D levels had either a lower incidence of colon cancer or decreased mortality. Similarly, 9 of the 13 studies about breast cancer and 13 of the 26 studies about prostate cancer showed beneficial effects of vitamin D levels on cancer incidence or mortality.** (Garland et al, 2006)

A 2007 population-based randomized, control trial found that **post-menopausal women who were supplemented with calcium** and vitamin D had a reduced risk of cancer after the first year of treatment. (Lappe et al, 2007)

Very recently, Northwestern University researchers said that vitamin D can help reduce the risk of aggressive prostate cancer in men.

Cancer patients who have higher levels of vitamin D when they are diagnosed tend to have better survival rates and remain in remission longer than patients who are vigtamin D-deficient. (Journal of Clinical Endocrinology & Metabolism (JCEM), 2014)

A new 2014 study published in the journal *Clinical Cancer Research* suggests that vitamin D deficiency may be an indicator of aggressive prostate cancer.

Vitamin D summary condensed facts

The following condensed facts were excerpted from the article by Grober et al, 2013.

- According to recent studies, a vitamin D deficiency [serum 25(OH)D <20 ng/mL] is likely to be an important etiological factor in the pathogenesis of many chronic diseases. These include autoimmune diseases (e.g., multiple sclerosis, type I diabetes) inflammatory bowel disease (e.g., Crohn disease), infections (such as infections of the upper respiratory tract), immune deficiency, cardiovascular diseases (e.g., hypertension, heart failure, sudden cardiac death), cancer (e.g., colon cancer, breast cancer, non-Hodgkin's lymphoma) and neurocognitive disorders (e.g., Alzheimer disease)

- Vitamin D deficiency is common in cancer patients and correlates with disease progression. In observational studies, vitamin D deficiency is associated with increased incidence of breast and colon cancer as well as with an unfavorable course of non-Hodgkin lymphoma. (Churilla et al, 2012)

- In breast cancer patients under polychemotherapy with anthracycline and taxane, a significant drop in 25(OH)D levels was observed. (Santini et al, 2010)

- The vitamin D hormone has a significant impact on the cardiovascular system, central nervous system, endocrine system and immune system as well as on cell differentiation and cell growth.

- **Vitamin D plays an important role in the calcium and phosphorus metabolism and helps ensure adequate levels of these minerals for metabolic functions and bone mineralization**

- The **Intermountain Heart Collaborative Study, a prospective study with 41,504 participants,** an inadequate vitamin D supply was determined in 63.6% [25(OH)D: < 30 ng/mL). **A 25(OH)D level <15 ng/mL compared with a 25(OH)D levels >30 ng/mL was associated with a highly significant increase in the prevalence of type 2 diabetes, high blood pressure, dyslipoproteinaemia, peripheral vascular diseases, coronary heart disease, myocardial infarction, cardiac insufficiency and stroke as well as in the incidence of overall mortality, cardiac insufficiency, coronary heart disease / myocardial infarction, stroke, and their combination.** (Anderson et al, 2010)

- That 25(OH)D levels ≤12.4 ng/ml compared with 25(OH)D levels of >18.8 ng/ml **was associated with an increase in the risk level for strokes of 53%.** (Sun et al, 2012)

- **A deficiency of vitamin D [25(OH)D <20 ng/mL or 50 nmol/L] significantly increases overall and cardiovascular mortality.** (Dobnig et al, 2008)

- **A vitamin D deficiency significantly increased general and cardiovascular mortality over a follow up median of 9.5 years. (the ESTHER study,** a nationwide cohort study**)**

- **Vitamin D deficiency was also associated with significantly increased cancer mortality and a higher mortality rate for respiratory diseases -** (Schottker et al, 2013)

- **A systematic review and a meta-analysis conclude that vitamin D lowers systolic blood pressure by −6.18 mmHg and reduces diastolic blood pressure by -3.1 mmHg in hypertensive patients.** No change in blood pressure was observed in normotensive persons. (Witham et al, 2009)

- **Newborn babies who receive 2000 IU of vitamin D$_3$ daily as rickets prophylaxis showed a 88% lower risk for type 1 diabetes mellitus compared with those with lower-dosed** supplementation. The risk for type 1 diabetes in infants who received a vitamin D supplement compared with those who received no vitamin D was reduced by 29%. (Zipitis et al, 2008)

- A low maternal 25(OH)D status (≤54 nmol/L or 21.6 ng/mL) during pregnancy was associated with a more than 2-fold risk increase for the development of type 1 diabetes later in life compared with a good maternal 25(OH)D status (>89 nmol/L or 35.6 ng/mL). (Sorensen et al, 2012)

- In a meta-analysis of 16 studies, the odds ratio for type 2 diabetes was 1.50 (1.33–1.70) for the bottom vs top quartile of 25(OH)D. (Afzal et al, 2013)

- In Australian adults vitamin D deficiency [25(OH)D <20 ng/mL] and vitamin D insufficiency [25-OH-D: 21–29 ng/mL] were associated with a significantly increased risk for metabolic syndrome ($P < 0.01$), insulin resistance, high waist circumference and raised glucose and triglyceride levels. (Gagnon et al, 2012)

- A recent systematic review and meta-analysis of 11 randomized controlled trials with 5,660 patients vitamin D showed a protective effect against respiratory tract infections (RTIs). The protective effect was larger in studies using once-daily dosing compared with bolus doses. (Bergman et al, 2013)

- The risk of influenza A was reduced in Japanese school children by the supplementation of vitamin D_3 by 42%. (Urashima et al, 2010)

- Vitamin D and its analogs are playing an increasing role in the management of atopic dermatitis, psoriasis, vitiligo, acne and rosacea. (Youssef et al, 2011)

- The association of vitamin D deficiency with markers of disease activity in rheumatoid arthritis (RA) present mixed results.

-There is no doubt about the important role vitamin D plays in the development and progression of MS. (Ho et al, 2012)

- In older individuals vitamin D deficiency is associated with an increased risk of functional limitations, falling and fractures. (Hollick et al, 2012) (Sohl et al, 2013)

- Recent meta-analysis from 11 **double-blind and randomized studies showed a statistically non-significant reduction of hip fractures by 10%.** (Bischoff-Ferrari et al, 2012)

- **Significant reduction in the risk of falling is already observed after 2–3 mo of vitamin D supplementation.** (Bischoff-Ferrari et al, 2009a)

- **Vitamin D is important for dental health and a promising factor in the prevention of caries.** (Hujoel, 2013)

- **Although navy personnel who were outside all the time were 8 times more likely to develop skin cancer compared with age-matched controls who work indoors they had a 60% reduced risk of dying of cancer than the civilian population.** (Pellar, Stephensen, 1937)

- **Grant reported a dramatic inverse relationship between premature mortality due to cancer with UV exposure in both men and women.** (Grant, 2002)

- **A meta-analysis of cancer incidence rates for more than 100 countries concluded that there was an inverse relationship with solar UVB exposure for 15 types of cancers including endometrial, gastric, cervical, bladder, pancreatic and colorectal cancer among others.** (Grant, 2012)

- **Women who had the most sun exposure as teenagers and young adults had a more than 60% reduced risk of developing breast cancer.** (Knight et al, 2007)

- **A similar observation with prostate cancer in men who worked outdoors; these men had a 3 y hiatus before developing prostate cancer** compared with indoor workers. (Luscombe et al, 2001)

- **A prospective study in men and found an inverse association with cancer incidence of GI related cancers and predictors of vitamin D status.** (Giovannucci et al, 2006)

- **A large number of publications have related increased sun exposure, living at lower latitudes and increased vitamin D intake with reduced risk not only for cancers but also autoimmune diseases including type 1 diabetes, rheumatoid arthritis, and multiple sclerosis, neurological disorders including** depression and schizophrenia, infectious diseases including tuberculosis and lower blood pressure.

- living for the first 10 years of your life below 35° north and above 35° south latitude reduces risk for developing multiple sclerosis by 50%. (Grant, 2010)

- **Being born and living near the equator reduces risk of type 1 diabetes by more than 10-fold compared with living in the far northern and southern regions of the globe**. (Mohr et al, 2008)

- Higher latitude (Northern hemisphere) and lower latitude (Southern hemisphere) has been linked to more high blood pressure, and greater risk for schizophrenia and higher risk for tuberculosis.

Since the Grober article was a review article, I decided to include a modified version of it, although it appears to be a selective "positive" review. It follows:

Vitamin D: Update 2013: From rickets prophylaxis to general preventive healthcare

Abstract

Vitamin D has received a lot of attention recently as a result of **a meteoric rise** in the number of publications showing that vitamin D plays a crucial role in a plethora of physiological functions and **associating vitamin D deficiency with many acute and chronic illnesses including disorders of calcium metabolism, autoimmune diseases, some cancers, type 2 diabetes mellitus, infectious diseases and cardiovascular disease**. The recent data on vitamin D from experimental, ecological, case-control, retrospective and prospective observational studies, as well as smaller intervention studies, are significant and **confirm the sunshine vitamin's essential role in a variety of physiological and preventative functions**. The results of **these studies justify the recommendation to improve the general vitamin D status in children and adults by means of a healthy approach to sunlight exposure, consumption of**

foods containing vitamin D and supplementation with vitamin D preparations. In general, closer attention should therefore be paid to vitamin D deficiency in medical and pharmaceutical practice than has been the case hitherto. (Grober et al, 2013)

Introduction

Since the discovery of its antirachitic effect in the 1920s, the sunshine vitamin was for many years only seen in relation to its function in calcium and bone metabolism. A variety of research results from recent years have shown that vitamin D in its hormonally active form, $1\alpha,25$-dihydroxyvitamin D [$1\alpha,25(OH)_2D$; calcitriol] is not only a regulator of calcium and phosphate homeostasis, but has numerous extra-skeletal effects. These include the significant impact of the vitamin D hormone on the cardiovascular system, central nervous system, endocrine system and immune system as well as on cell differentiation and cell growth.

$1\alpha,25(OH)_2D$ manifests its diverse biological effects (endocrine, autocrine, paracrine) by binding to the vitamin D receptor (VDR) found in most body cells. Vitamin D receptors have been found in over 35 target tissues that are not involved in bone metabolism. These include endothelial cells, islet cells of the pancreas, hematopoietic cells, cardiac and skeletal muscle cells, monocytes, neurons, placental cells and T-lymphocytes. It is estimated that VDR activation may regulate directly and/or indirectly a very large number of genes (0.5–5% of the total human genome i.e., 100–1250 genes). The fact that the vitamin D receptor is expressed by many tissues results in the pronounced pleiotropic effect of vitamin D hormone.

From Sunshine Vitamin to Sunshine Hormone

Vitamin D—the sunshine vitamin—is formed in the skin from 7-dehydrocholesterol (7-DHC) via the intermediate previtamin D_3 and with the help of sunlight (UVB: 290–315 nm). Previtamin D_3 is converted by body heat to vitamin D_3[cholecalciferol]. Excessive sunlight exposure degrades previtamin D_3 and vitamin D_3 to inactive photoproducts, thus preventing excessive production of the sunshine vitamin in the skin. The liver converts vitamin D_3 via the enzyme 25-hydroxylase (25-OHase: CYP27A1, CYP2R1) into **25-hydroxyvitamin D [25(OH)D], also known as calcidiol**. The mitochondrial CYP27A1 and microsomal CYP2R1 are the two major enzymes involved in the hydroxylation at C-25, although there are several CYP enzymes that show 25-hydroxylase (25-OHase) activity but with higher K_m and lower V_{max}.. **Serum 25(OH)D (1 ng/mL = 2,5 nmol/L) is the barometer for the medical laboratory evaluation of the vitamin D status.**

25(OH)D is then converted in the kidneys via the enzyme 25-hydroxyvitamin D-1-α-hydroxylase also known as cytochrome p450 27B1 (1-OHase: CYP27B1) into the metabolically active vitamin D hormone [1α,25(OH)$_2$D]. This enzyme is also called *renal 1-α-hydroxylase* - since it occurs in the kidneys (→ **endocrine effect**). The renal synthesis of 1,25(OH)$_2$D is regulated by several factors including serum phosphorus, calcium, fibroblast growth factor 23 (FGF-23), parathyroid hormone (PTH) and itself. Besides the kidneys, a multitude of tissues have a local 1-α-hydroxylase (1-OHase) including bone, placenta, prostate, keratinocytes, macrophages, T-lymphocytes, dendritic cells, several cancer cells, and the parathyroid gland.

Depending on the availability of 25(OH)D and the amounts required, these cells can produce the biologically active vitamin D hormone with the help of their local 1-OHase (→ autocrine and paracrine effect). **1α,25(OH)$_2$D is like the sex hormones (e.g., estradiol) and corticosteroids (e.g., cortisone), which are all steroid hormones.**

Via a feedback mechanism, the 1α,25(OH)$_2$D level regulates the synthesis of 1α,25(OH)$_2$D and reduces the synthesis and secretion of parathyroid hormone in the parathyroid glands. 1α,25(OH)$_2$D induces its own destruction by activating the 25-hydroxyvitamin D-24-hydroxylase (24-OHase: CYP24A1), which leads to the multistep catabolism of both 25(OH)D and 1α,25(OH)$_2$D into biologically inactive, water-soluble metabolites including calcitroic acid.

The Barometer of Vitamin D Health: 25-hydroxyvitamin D

According to current scientific knowledge, the serum 25(OH)D level should be between 30 and 100 ng/mL to avoid long-term negative health consequences.

A 25(OH)D status between 40 and 60 ng/mL or 100 to 150 nmol/L is ideal.

A pronounced vitamin D deficiency is present at 25(OH)D levels below 20 ng/mL, with levels between 21–29 ng/mL designated as moderate vitamin D deficiency, also referred to as vitamin D insufficiency.

Vitamin D intoxication is only to be expected at levels of 25(OH)D > 150 ng/mL.

Vitamin D deficiency is often accompanied with elevation in serum parathyroid hormone (PTH) levels. Evidence is increasing that PTH elevation may promote cardiovascular disease through diminished cardiac contractility, enhanced coronary risk, and cardiac valvular and vascular calcification.

The high proportion of blood samples showing a vitamin D deficiency and secondary hyperparathyroidism was remarkable in this analysis. Active $1,25(OH)_2D$ should not be measured to assess vitamin D status, since in the presence of a vitamin D deficiency it is often normal or even shows a compensatory increase due to elevated parathyroid hormone levels!

North of the 35th parallel, the sun is not high enough in the sky from October to March to supply our skin with the necessary 290 to 315 nm UVB radiation. The flat angle of incidence of the sun is responsible for the low intensity of the sun's rays. Germany is located between 47th and 55th parallels, i.e., in the northern hemisphere of the earth, at same level as Canada. This also explains why so many people, especially in the winter months, suffer from vitamin D deficiency [25(OH) D <20 ng/mL or 50 nmol/L]. The UV index can also be used to estimate sun-dependent vitamin D formation in the skin. **With a UV index of less than 3, no vitamin D synthesis can take place in the skin.**

An App for the iPhone*dminder.info* provides the user anywhere on the planet information about how much vitamin D can be made in the skin during sun exposure. **Vitamin D intake in the diet plays only a minor role in the vitamin D supply.**

Based on the results of recent studies, approximately 1 billion people worldwide are affected by a vitamin D deficiency [25-OH-D: <20 ng/mL] or a vitamin D insufficiency [25(OH) D: 21–29 ng/mL].

Health Risk: Vitamin D Deficiency

According to recent studies, a vitamin D deficiency [serum 25(OH)D <20 ng/mL] is likely to be an important etiological factor in the pathogenesis of many chronic diseases. These include autoimmune diseases (e.g., multiple sclerosis, type I diabetes) inflammatory bowel disease (e.g., Crohn disease), infections (such as infections of the upper respiratory tract), immune deficiency, cardiovascular diseases (e.g., hypertension, heart failure, sudden cardiac death), cancer (e.g., colon cancer, breast cancer, non-Hodgkin's lymphoma) and neurocognitive disorders (e.g., Alzheimer disease).

The current results of the **ESTHER study**, a nationwide cohort study from the Saarland, involving about 10,000 women and men aged 50 to 74 years in whom the 25(OH)D status was ascertained, showed that **a vitamin D deficiency significantly increased general and cardiovascular mortality over a follow up median of 9.5 years**. The 25(OH)D levels and overall mortality showed a pronounced nonlinear inverse association with increased risk beginning at 25(OH)D levels below 75 nmol/l (<30 ng/ml).

A vitamin D deficiency was also associated with significantly increased cancer mortality and a higher mortality rate for respiratory diseases. (Schottker et al, 2013))

Bone, Muscle Metabolism, and Dental Health: Fractures, Falls and Caries

Vitamin D plays an important role in the calcium and phosphorus metabolism and helps ensure adequate levels of these minerals for metabolic functions and bone mineralization. $1\alpha,25(OH)_2D$ increases the efficiency of intestinal calcium absorption from 10–15% to 30–40% by interacting with the VDR-RXR and thereby promoting the expression of an epithelial calcium channel and a calcium-binding protein.

A severe vitamin D deficiency [25(OH)D <10 ng/mL] results in rickets in children and osteomalacia in adults. The clinical symptoms of a severe vitamin D deficiency include, besides a mineralization disorder, a myopathy with proximal muscle weakness and muscle pain. The mineralization disorder osteomalacia can also cause bone pain and fractures.

In older individuals vitamin D deficiency is associated with an increased risk of functional limitations, falling and fractures. (Hollick et al, 2012) (Sohl et al, 2013)

These data shed a new light on the impact of vitamin D deficiency in bone health and explains why **a normal vitamin D status is essential to maintain bone's structural integrity.**[16]

In the most recent meta-analysis original data on 30,011 study participants from **11 double-blind and randomized studies** were pooled. The classic intent-to-treat analysis of 30,011 persons **showed a statistically non-significant reduction of hip fractures by 10%.** (Bischoff-Ferrari et al, 2012)

However, an analysis of the effect in relation to the vitamin D amount actually taken, showed a statistically significant reduction of hip fractures by 30% among the subjects taking the highest dosage (792 to 2000 IU vitamin D/day; median: 800 IU vitamin D/day) compared with the control group. **In persons supplemented with less than 792 IU vitamin D per day, no statistically significant reduction of hip fractures was detectable.** A similar dose-effect dependence was detected for all non-vertebral fractures. **The subgroup analysis showed a significant reduction of fractures in all age groups, for elderly people living at home as well as those living in nursing homes with the highest vitamin D dosage.** (Bischoff-Ferrari et al, 2012)

The results of a bone biopsy study of 675 presumed healthy adults aged 20 to 90 years, who died in an accident indicated a threshold level of 25(OH)D ≥75 nmol/L or ≥30 ng/mL as a target value for healthy bone metabolism at which further no mineralization disorder (osteomalacia) was detected.

In addition to a positive effect on bone mineral density, **vitamin D has an immediate restorative effect on the muscles**, which can be explained in terms of a better influx of calcium into the muscle cells as well as a receptor-mediated stimulation of muscle protein synthesis.[18,19] It may be that this additional effect is a crucial factor in the fracture reduction observed with vitamin D supplementation, since falling represents the primary risk factor for fractures. This is also supported by study results according to which **a significant reduction in the risk of falling is already observed after 2–3 mo of vitamin D**

supplementation, indicating that the musculature responds quite rapidly to vitamin D intake, and fracture reduction is noticeable after only about 6 mo. (Bischoff-Ferrari et al, 2009)

In the reanalysis of a meta-analysis of 8 double-blind and randomized studies, which had been published in 2009, with high-quality detection of the factor falling, **vitamin D demonstrated a benefit in all studies**. The relevance of vitamin D dosing with respect to reduction of falls could also be confirmed: at the higher dose (700–1000 IU vitamin D/day), vitamin D reduced the risk of a fall by 34%, while no reduction of falls was observed at the lower dosage level).(Bischoff-Ferrari et al, 2011)

In addition to the crucial role of vitamin D for bone health several studies have shown an association between alveolar bone density, osteoporosis and tooth loss. Low bone mass may be a risk factor for periodontal disease. A recent systematic review and meta-analysis of controlled clinical trials indicate that **vitamin D is important for dental health and a promising factor in the prevention of caries**. This could be due to the fact that vitamin D has a direct effect on bone metabolism and can also act as an anti-inflammatory agent and stimulate the production of anti-microbial peptides. (Hujoel, 2013)

Comment: Improvement in 25(OH)D status by supplementation with vitamin D_2 or vitamin D_3 is an important health strategy to promote bone health at all age levels and to reduce the risk of fractures and falling in the elderly. To maximize the osseous effect and intestinal calcium absorption, supplementation should achieve a 25(OH)D status of ≥75 nmol/l or ≥30 ng/ml.

Ecological Association Studies

Over the past 100 years there have been a variety of ecological studies that have associated living at higher latitudes with many acute and chronic illnesses. One of the first association studies was reported by Palm in 1889 when he realized that children living in the inner cities of Great Britain were at extremely high risk for developing the devastating bone deforming disease rickets while children living in India had little evidence for the disease. He was one of the first to recommend sunbathing for promoting skeletal health and reducing risk for rickets.

In 1921 Hess and Unger reported that sun exposure was effective in treating and preventing rickets.

The relationship between sun exposure, rickets and vitamin D$_3$ was finally appreciated in the early 1930s when Windaus determined that vitamin D$_3$ was produced in mammalian skin and was identified as the antirachtic factor by many investigators.

One of the first ecological studies relating latitude and cancer was reported by Hoffman in 1916. He observed that **cancer mortality between 1908 and 1912 was increased in people living at higher latitudes**. Peller and Stephensen reported on the incidence of cancer in navy personnel in the United States and noted that **although navy personnel who were outside all the time were 8 times more likely to develop skin cancer compared with age-matched controls who work indoors they had a 60% reduced risk of dying of cancer than the civilian population**. (Pellar, Stephensen, 1937)

This was followed by Apperly who in 1941 reported total cancer mortality in Americans and Canadians in the same population who were engaged in agriculture. He concluded that **cancer mortality was highest in farmers living in the northeast compared with those living in the south.**

In the 1980s through the early 2000s there were several reports of associations with increased risk for colon, ovarian, prostate cancer and many other cancers for people living at higher latitudes in the United States as well as in Europe.

Grant reported a dramatic inverse relationship between premature mortality due to cancer with UV exposure in both men and women. (Grant, 2002)

A meta-analysis of cancer incidence rates for more than 100 countries including Australia, and China among others confirm previous studies where it was concluded that there was an inverse relationship with solar UVB exposure for 15 types of cancers including endometrial, gastric, cervical, bladder, pancreatic and colorectal cancer among others. (Grant, 2012)

Not only the relative risk for developing deadly cancers was associated with less solar UVB exposure but also mortality from these numerous malignancies was also related to less solar UVB exposure.

A study conducted in Canada reported that women who had the most sun exposure as teenagers and young adults had a more than 60% reduced risk of developing breast cancer

compared with women living in the same locale who had minimum sun exposure during the same period of time. (Knight et al, 2007)

Luscombe et al. made a **similar observation with prostate cancer in men who worked outdoors; these men had a 3 y hiatus before developing prostate cancer** compared with indoor workers. (Luscombe et al, 2001)

The connection between increased sun exposure and living at lower latitudes with reduced risk for cancers with vitamin D was first described by Garland and Garland. They first related a strong significant negative correlation with colon cancer and mortality with mean daily radiation in the United States. This was followed by an 8 y prospective case-controlled study of adults living in Washington County where the risk of developing colon cancer was reduced 3-fold in people who had a baseline 25(OH)D >20 ng/mL.

Giovannucci et al. conducted **a prospective study in men and found an inverse association with cancer incidence of GI related cancers and predictors of vitamin D status.** (Giovannucci et al, 2006)

These studies have been followed by **a large number of publications that have related increased sun exposure, living at lower latitudes and increased vitamin D intake with reduced risk not only for cancers but also autoimmune diseases including type 1 diabetes, rheumatoid arthritis, and multiple sclerosis, neurological disorders including depression and schizophrenia, infectious diseases including tuberculosis and lower blood pressure.**

Evidence suggests that **living for the first 10 years of your life below 35° north and above 35° south latitude reduces risk for developing multiple sclerosis by 50%.** (Grant, 2010)

Being born and living near the equator reduces risk of type 1 diabetes by more than 10-fold compared with living in the far northern and southern regions of the globe. (Mohr et al, 2008)

Women living at higher latitudes in the US were at higher risk for developing rheumatoid arthritis. **People in Scandinavia are more likely to develop schizophrenia compared with people living near the equator and babies born at the end of the winter are more likely to develop schizophrenia even those born in Australia.** Patients with TB were found to do better when exposed to sunlight and curiously it was known that **living in the Alps above 5,000 feet the incidence of TB was very low.**

Finally, **it was demonstrated that the higher the latitude that you live in the northern hemisphere and the lower the latitude that you live in the southern hemisphere, was associated with a higher overall blood pressure.**

Many of these ecologic observations which suggest a direct role of increased sun exposure and improved vitamin D status has been supported by association and prospective and retrospective studies relating vitamin D intake or vitamin D status with these chronic illnesses.

Gene Expression: Link Between Vitamin D and Prevention

In a recent **randomized, placebo-controlled, double-blind study**, the influence of a daily supplementation of 400 IU or 2000 IU of vitamin D_3 over a period of two months in winter on the gene expression of white blood cells (leukocytes) in healthy adults was investigated for the first time. **The improvement of 25(OH)D status observed thereby was associated with a change in gene expression of at least 1.5-fold in 291 genes.** The results of this study suggest that **any improvement in vitamin D status will significantly affect the expression of genes.**

Cardiovascular System: Hypertension and Cardiac Insufficiency

A deficiency of vitamin D [25(OH)D <20 ng/mL or 50 nmol/L] significantly increases overall and cardiovascular mortality. (Dobnig et al, 2008)

In the **Intermountain Heart Collaborative Study, a prospective study with 41,504 participants**, an inadequate vitamin D supply was determined in 63.6% [25(OH)D: < 30 ng/mL). **A 25(OH)D level <15 ng/mL compared with a 25(OH)D levels >30 ng/mL was associated with a highly significant increase in the prevalence of type 2 diabetes, high blood pressure, dyslipoproteinaemia,** peripheral vascular diseases, coronary heart disease, myocardial infarction, cardiac insufficiency and stroke as well as in the incidence of overall mortality, cardiac insufficiency, coronary heart disease / myocardial infarction, stroke, and their combination. (Anderson et al, 2010)

The results of a meta-analysis covering the vitamin D status with the risk for cerbrovascular events, including >1200 cases of stroke, revealed that 25(OH)D levels ≤12.4 ng/ml compared with 25(OH)D levels of >18.8 ng/ml was associated with an increase in the risk level for strokes of 53%. (Sun et al, 2012)

A systematic review and a meta-analysis conclude that vitamin D lowers systolic blood pressure by –6.18 mmHg and reduces diastolic blood pressure by -3.1 mmHg in hypertensive patients. No change in blood pressure was observed in normotensive persons. (Witham et al, 2009)

Black US. Americans suffer significantly more frequently from high blood pressure than whites. Darker skin color generally produce less vitamin D_3 in the skin due to the higher content of melanin and thus have lower levels of 25(OH)D. For each increase of 25(OH)D levels by 1 ng/ml, a significant reduction in systolic blood pressure of 0.2 mmHg was detected. However, no significant reduction in diastolic blood pressure was detected.

In another 16-week randomized clinical trial with normotensive black boys and girls the relation between 25(OH)D concentrations and total body fat mass by dual-energy X-ray absorptiometry, and the arterial stiffness measured by pulse wave velocity (PWV) in response to 2000 IU vitamin D supplementation was analyzed. The results demonstrate that vitamin D supplementation may be effective in optimizing vitamin D status and counteracting the progression of aortic stiffness in black youth. Plasma 25(OH)D concentrations in response to the 2000 IU/d supplementation were negatively influenced by adiposity.

The suppression of parathyroid hormone (PTH) by vitamin D, which has been known for some time, must now be seen in a new light, since PTH has been increasingly recognized in recent years as a major risk factor for cardiovascular diseases such as high blood pressure or cardiac insufficiency. In addition, vitamin D counteracts the adverse effects of the so-called "advanced glycation endproducts" (AGEs) on the endothelium.

In a recent placebo-controlled, double-blind study of 80 infants with cardiac insufficiency, daily supplementation of 1200 IU vitamin D3 for a period of 12 weeks in the 42 children from the vitamin D group compared with the 38 children in the placebo group resulted in a significant improvement in the performance of the heart muscle (e.g., LVEF ↑) and the reduction of various cardiovascular risk parameters.

Another recent study evaluated the effect of vitamin D insufficiency (< 30 ng/mL) on epicardial coronary flow rate, subclinical atherosclerosis, and endothelial function in 222 consecutive patients who had undergone coronary angiography for suspected ischemic heart disease and were found to have normal or near-normal coronary arteries. The mean level of 25(OH)D was 31.8 ng/ml, and 47% (n = 106) of the patients had insufficient 25(OH)D levels (<30 ng/ml). Baseline characteristics were similar between vitamin D insufficient and vitamin D sufficient groups. **The incidence of slow coronary flow (SCF) was significantly higher in the vitamin D insufficient group than in patients with sufficient vitamin D.** After adjusting for cardiovascular disease risk factors, **VD insufficiency was independently associated with SCF.** The linear regression analysis showed that VD insufficiency was correlated independently with % flow-mediated dilatation and carotid intima-media thickness.

Diabetology

Type I diabetes

The worldwide incidence rate of type I diabetes is increasing and accumulating data show that it is associated with vitamin D deficiency. The chronic autoimmune disease type I diabetes usually results from a T cell mediated destruction of insulin producing, pancreatic β-cells with a typical onset in childhood or adolescence. **There is evidence that vitamin D supplementation early in life is a protective factor against the development of type I diabetes.** Furthermore, in animal models, such as the NOD mice, the administration of $1\alpha,25(OH)_2D$ or vitamin D analogs prevented or at least delayed the onset of diabetes.

In a Finnish cohort study involving 12,058 children, the influence of supplementation of vitamin D in the first year of life on incidence of diabetes was followed up over a period of 30 y. It was found that **newborn**

babies who receive 2000 IU of vitamin D$_3$ daily as rickets prophylaxis showed a 88% lower risk for type 1 diabetes mellitus compared with those with lower-dosed supplementation. Children who suffered from rickets in the first year of life had a 3-fold higher risk for type 1 diabetes compared with healthy children.[66] In a meta-analysis of 4 case-control studies, **the risk for type 1 diabetes in infants who received a vitamin D supplement compared with those who received no vitamin D was reduced by 29%.** (Zipitis et al, 2008)

The importance of maternal vitamin D status on subsequent development of type 1 diabetes in newborns is described by a Norwegian cohort study of 20 072 women. **A low maternal 25(OH)D status (≤54 nmol/L or 21.6 ng/mL) during pregnancy was associated with a more than 2-fold risk increase for the development of type 1 diabetes later in life** compared with a good maternal 25(OH)D status (>89 nmol/L or 35.6 ng/mL). (Sorensen et al, 2012)

Type 2 diabetes and metabolic syndrome

Vitamin D deficiency has been implicated in decreased insulin secretion and increased insulin resistance, hallmarks of type 2 diabetes mellitus. The results of a recent published prospective cohort study and meta-analysis with 9,841 participants of whom 810 developed type 2 diabetes during a 29 years follow-up confirm once more an association of low 25(OH)D serum levels with an increased risk of type 2 diabetes. **Lower 25(OH)D concentrations were associated with higher cumulative incidence of type 2 diabetes.** Multivariable adjusted hazard ratios of type 2 diabetes were 1.22 for 25(OH)D <5 vs ≥20 µg/L and 1.35 for lowest vs highest quartile.

Finally, **in a meta-analysis of 16 studies, the odds ratio for type 2 diabetes was 1.50 (1.33–1.70) for the bottom vs top quartile of 25(OH)D.** (Afzal et al, 2013)

In a randomized, placebo-controlled study involving insulin-resistant South Asian women (age: 23–68 years) with median 25(OH)D baseline levels of <10 ng/ml, daily supplementation of 4,000 IU vitamin D$_3$ led to a significant improvement in insulin sensitivity and reduction of insulin resistance compared with placebo.

Several studies showed an inverse correlation of 25(OH)D concentration with metabolic syndrome risk or with the incidence or severity of its components.

Subjects with hypovitaminosis D are at higher risk of insulin resistance and the metabolic syndrome. The association of 25(OH)D level with the incidence of metabolic syndrome was analyzed in 4,164 Australian adults (age ±50 years) in a recent prospective study. They concluded that **in Australian adults vitamin D deficiency [25(OH)D <20 ng/mL] and vitamin D insufficiency [25-OH-D: 21–29 ng/mL] were associated with a significantly increased risk for metabolic syndrome ($P < 0.01$), insulin resistance, high waist circumference and raised glucose and triglyceride levels.** (Gagnon et al, 2012)

The results of a further prospective study provide additional meaningful results in support of the thesis that a vitamin D deficiency accelerates the progression of pre-diabetes to manifest type 2 diabetes.

Respiratory tract diseases (RTI)

A series of observational and epidemiological studies, supported by interventional studies and the ubiquitous evidence of vitamin D receptors in all major organ systems, show an association between 25(OH)D levels and a reduced incidence of infections of the upper respiratory system.

In a recent systematic review and meta-analysis of 11 randomized controlled trials with 5,660 patients vitamin D showed a protective effect against respiratory tract infections (RTIs). The protective effect was larger in studies using once-daily dosing compared with bolus doses. (Bergman et al, 2013)

In a recent randomized double-blinded trial with 247 Mongolian schoolchildren the effect of daily ingestion of vitamin D unfortified or fortified milk (fortified with 300 IU vitamin D) was evaluated. At baseline, the median serum 25(OH)D level was 7 ng/mL. **Vitamin D supplementation significantly reduced the risk of ARIs in winter among Mongolian children with vitamin D deficiency.**

In a randomized, placebo-controlled, double-blind study of 334 Japanese schoolchildren, the influence of vitamin D_3 supplementation on respiratory diseases such as influenza A and asthma was investigated. The children received a placebo or 1200 IU vitamin D_3 daily during the intervention period from December 2008 to March 2009. **The risk of influenza A was reduced by the supplementation of vitamin D_3 by 42%** compared with placebo. The protective effect was particularly pronounced in the children who took no other vitamin D-containing supplements. The result in relation to the frequency of asthma attacks is even more impressive: In the vitamin D group, the frequency of asthma attacks decreased by 83%. (Urashima et al, 2010)

Also in interventional studies with adults, the supplementation of vitamin D_3 led to a significant reduction in seasonal flu-like infections.

Atopic dermatitis, psoriasis other dermatides

The ability of vitamin D to regulate local immune and inflammatory responses offers exciting potential for understanding and treating chronic inflammatory dermatitides. That is why **vitamin D and its analogs are playing an increasing role in the management of atopic dermatitis, psoriasis, vitiligo, acne and rosacea.** (Youssef et al, 2011)

Vitamin D hormone [$1,25(OH)_2D$] has a pronounced modulating effect on the balance between the Th1 and Th-2 cells. Th1:Th2 imbalances play a pathogenic role in atopic disease in addition to autoimmune diseases such as multiple sclerosis. In two randomized, placebo-controlled, double-blind studies of vitamin D supplementation only (1,600 IU / day, PO) and in combination with vitamin E (600 IU/ day, PO) over a period of 60 d led to significant improvement of skin findings in patients (age: 13–45 years of age) with mild, moderate, and severe atopic dermatitis. To assess the extent and intensity of atopic eczema, the SCORAD score (Scoring Atopic Dermatitis) was used. In atopic dermatitis, the inflammatory processes in the skin are associated with an intensive infiltration of lymphocytes and eosinophils, **which release proinflammatory cytokines, superoxide radicals, hydrogen peroxides and peroxynitrite.** Remarkably, these studies demonstrated that not only vitamin E, but also vitamin D reduces the oxidative load and inflammatory processes in the skin and **significantly increases the activity level of the erythrocytic superoxide dismutase (SOD) and catalase (CAT).** (Javanbakht et al, 2010)

Autoimmune disease: rheumatoid arthritis, IBD and multiple sclerosis

In addition to infectious diseases Vitamin D plays a contributory role in the pathophysiology of autoimmune diseases. This is further supported by various experimental findings showing vitamin D's capability to regulate chemokine production, counteracting autoimmune inflammation and to induce differentiation of immune cells in a way that promotes self-tolerance.

The increased prevalence of auto-immune diseases at higher latitudes has been shown for multiple **sclerosis (MS), inflammatory bowel disease, rheumatoid arthritis and type I diabetes.**

Several studies have looked at the association of vitamin D deficiency with markers of disease activity in RA with somewhat mixed results.

In the Iowa Women's Health Study of 29,368 women of ages 55–69 years without a history of rheumatoid arthritis at study baseline showed **that greater intake (highest vs. lowest tertile) of vitamin D was inversely associated with the risk of rheumatoid arthritis.**

In contrast in a larger cohort of 186,389 women followed in **the Nurses Health Studies there was no correlation between serum levels of Vitamin D and later development of RA.**

On the other hand recently an evaluation of in vitro effects of $1\alpha,25(OH)_2D_3$ in primary cultures of peripheral blood monocyte-derived macrophages of RA patients and healthy subjects was reported.

Nonetheless, current evidence suggests that improving 25(OH)D status and/or using vitamin D receptor agonists may be useful in the treatment of inflammatory bowel disease and multiple sclerosis.

Even though the autoimmune origin of multiple sclerosis (MS) is increasingly discussed **there is no doubt about the important role vitamin D plays in the development and progression of MS.** (Ho et al, 2012)

Recent studies have shown that vitamin D deficiency may intensify traumatic brain injury and reduce the effects of other therapies for TBI.

Cancers

A large body of evidence indicates that solar UV-B (UVB) ir-radiance and vitamin D reduce the risk of incidence and death for many types of cancer.

For men, the UVB index was significantly inversely correlated with 14 types of internal cancer-bladder, breast, colon, gall-bladder, kidney, laryngeal, liver, lung, oral, pancreatic, pharyn-geal, prostate, rectal and small intestine cancer.

For women, the same UVB index was inversely correlated with bladder, breast and colon cancer. The results of many studies provide support for the UVB-vitamin D-cancer hypothesis and suggest that the widespread fear of chronic solar UV (UV) irradiance may be misplaced.

Vitamin D deficiency is common in cancer patients and cor-relates with disease progression. In observational studies, vi-tamin D deficiency is associated with increased incidence of breast and colon cancer as well as with an unfavorable course of non-Hodgkin lymphoma. (Churilla et al, 2012)

In a placebo-controlled, double-blind study of 1,179 postmenopausal women aged over 55 years, the influence of 1400 mg of calcium daily, the combination of 1,400 mg of calcium and 1100 I.U. of vitamin D_3 or placebo on the cancer risk was studied over a period of 4 years. In the woman who received the combination of calcium and vitamin D, the 25(OH)D level rose from 28.7 ng/mL to 38.4 ng/mL. Vitamin D status remained unchanged in the two other groups. **At the end of the four-year period, the relative risk (RR) of develop-ing cancer was reduced by 60% in the calcium + vitamin D_3 group as compared with the placebo group relative risk (RR) cancer, while in the group with calcium alone it was reduced by 47%.**

A reevaluation using logistic regression to cancer-free survival at 12 mo showed that the relative risk in the calcium + vita-min D_3 group had been significantly reduced by 77%. The data in the calcium group alone remained virtually unchanged. **Some studies indicate that the intake of vitamin D in the range of 1,100 to 4,000 IU/d and a 25(OH)D serum levels between 60 and 80 ng/ml may be needed to reduce the cancer risk.**

In a prospective cohort study, Canadian researchers from the Mount Sinai Hospital in Toronto observed the course of disease in 512 women with breast cancer for about 12 years from 1997 to 2008. The average age of the women was 50.4 years at diagnosis. 37.5 percent of the breast cancer patients had a vitamin D deficiency [25(OH)D <20 ng/mL or <50 nmol/L] when diagnosed. Only 24 percent of the affected women had an almost normal vitamin D status [25(OH)D > 29 ng/mL or 72 nmol/L]. **Vitamin D deficiency was associated with the occurrence of more aggressive forms of breast cancer. After 12 y, the risk of a metastasis in women with a vitamin D deficiency was increased by 94 percent compared with those with normal vitamin D status. The probability of premature death due to the disease rose in the presence of a vitamin D deficiency by 73 percent.**

In breast cancer patients under polychemotherapy with anthracycline and taxane, a significant drop in 25(OH)D levels was observed. (Santini et al, 2010)

Medical Drugs and Vitamin D

Drug-induced vitamin D imbalances must be reconsidered in the light of the high prophylactic potential of the sunshine vitamin. **It is known that many drugs can interfere with vitamin D metabolism.** Already in 1967 the association between osteomalacia and antiepileptic drug therapy was reported. Since then there have been many reports of abnormalities in calcium, vitamin D, and bone metabolism in subjects chronically treated not only with antiepileptic drugs but also with corticoids, rifampicin, and antiretroviral drugs. A drug-induced vitamin D deficiency [25(OH)D <20 ng/mL] may manifest as secondary hyperparathyroidism, bone mineralization disorders including the development of osteoporosis, and osteomalacia.

Treatment Strategies

Sensible sun exposure is the least expensive and most efficient way of obtaining an adequate amount of vitamin D. It has been estimated that a healthy adult in a bathing suit exposed to one minimal erythemal dose (MED) of sunlight is equivalent to ingesting about 20,000 IUs of vitamin D.

Thus the skin has a large capacity to produce vitamin D. Because time of day, season of the year and latitude along with degree of skin pigmentation has a dramatic effect on the cutaneous production of vitamin D there is no simple recommendation as to how much time to be exposed to obtain an adequate amount of vitamin D. However for example if a person knows that they are going to get a light pinkness to their skin 24 h later, i.e., a MED, by being exposed to 30 min of sun in their locale, the recommendation is to expose arms, legs and abdomen and back when possible for about 10–15 min followed by good sun protection.

Oral vitamin D (vitamin D_2 or D_3) can be taken on an empty stomach or with a meal. Both vitamin D_2 and vitamin D_3 at physiologic doses are effective in raising the blood level of 25(OH)D. The meal does not need to contain fat in order for the fat-soluble vitamin D to be absorbed. Furthermore vitamin D can be taken daily or the total amount can be taken once a week or even once a month as long as the total is the same i.e., 3000 IUs daily or 21 000 IUs weekly or 90 000 IUs monthly are equally effective in maintaining serum 25(OH)D levels in the desired range of 40–60 ng/mL.

To guarantee vitamin D sufficiency there are a variety of strategies to both treat and prevent vitamin D deficiency. One simple strategy that is effective is to fill the empty vitamin D tank with 50 000 IUs of vitamin D once a week for 8–12 weeks.

This is equivalent to ingesting approximately 6600 IUs daily. To prevent recurrence of vitamin D deficiency 50 000 IUs of vitamin D once every 2 weeks (equivalent to 3300 IUs daily) forever is effective in maintaining a healthy vitamin D status without causing toxicity.[142] Even young children have been effectively treated for vitamin D deficiency with 50 000 IUs of vitamin D weekly for 6 weeks or 2000 IUs of vitamin D daily.

Concluding Remarks

Closer attention should be paid to vitamin D deficiency in medical and pharmaceutical practice than has been the case hitherto. The data available to date on vitamin D from experimental, ecological, case-control, retrospective and prospective observational studies, as well as smaller

Prof Randolph M. Howes MD,PhD

intervention studies, are significant and confirm the sunshine vitamin's essential role in a variety of physiological and preventative functions, including neuropsychiatric disorders. The results of these studies justify the recommendation to improve the general vitamin D status in children and adults by means of a healthy approach to sunlight exposure, consumption of foods containing vitamin D and supplementation with vitamin D preparations. Nevertheless, **in a number of fields, we must await the results of controlled and randomized interventional studies involving the use of vitamin D in sufficiently high doses.** (Grober et al, 2013)

Received July 15, 2013; Revised October 7, 2013; Accepted October 8, 2013.

Vitamin D and its antioxidant analogues

Abstract

Vitamin D is a membrane antioxidant: thus Vitamin D3 (cholecalciferol) and its active metabolite 1,25-dihydroxycholecalciferol and also Vitamin D2 (ergocalciferol) and 7-dehydrocholesterol (pro-Vitamin D3) all inhibited iron-dependent liposomal lipid peroxidation. Cholecalciferol, 1,25-dihydroxycholecalciferol and ergocalciferol were **all of similar effectiveness as inhibitors of lipid peroxidation** but were less effective than 7-dehydrocholesterol; this was a better inhibitor of lipid peroxidation than cholesterol, though not ergosterol. The structural basis for the antioxidant ability of these Vitamin D compounds is considered in terms of their molecular relationship to cholesterol and ergosterol. Furthermore, the antioxidant ability of Vitamin D is compared to that of the anticancer drug tamoxifen and its 4-hydroxy metabolite (structural mimics of cholesterol) and discussed in relation to the anticancer action of this vitamin. (Wiseman, 1993)

Vitamin D and E stimulate SOD and CAT

The effects of vitamins E and D supplementation on erythrocyte superoxide dismutase and catalase in atopic dermatitis.

Abstract

BACKGROUND:

Atopic dermatitis is a public health problem worldwide. Increment of reactive oxygen species (ROS) production may be one of the contributing factors of tissue damage in atopic dermatitis. The present study was designed to determine the effect of vitamins E and/or D on erythrocyte superoxide dismutase and catalase activities in patients with atopic dermatitis.

METHODS:

In a **randomized, double blind, placebo controlled clinical trial 45 atopic dermatitis patients** were divided into four groups. Each group received one of the following supplements for 60 days: group A (n=11) vitamins E and D placebos; group B (n= 12) 1600 international unit (IU) vitamin D3 plus vitamin E placebo; group C (n=11) 600 IU synthetic all-rac-α tocopherol plus vitamin D placebo; group D (n=11) 1600 IU vitamin D3 plus 600 IU synthetic all-rac-α tocopherol. Erythrocyte superoxide dismutase (SOD) and catalase activities, serum 25 (OH) D, plasma α-tocopherol were determined. The data were analyzed by analysis of variance (ANOVA) and paired t-test.

RESULTS:

After 60 days vitamin D and E supplementation, erythrocyte SOD activities increased in groups B, C and D. Erythrocyte catalase activities increased in groups B and D. The increment of erythrocyte catalase activity was not significant in group C. **There was a positive significant correlation between SOD activity and serum 25 (OH) D**.

CONCLUSIONS:

It is concluded that **vitamin D is as potent as vitamin E in increasing the activities of erythrocyte SOD and catalase in atopic dermatitis patients.** (Javanbakht et al, 2010)

Prof Randolph M. Howes MD,PhD

Prooxidant nature of vitamin D

It must be kept in mind that vitamin D, like many other so-called anti-oxidants, has considerable prooxidant activity. This must be viewed in accordance with my voluminous other writings and I refer you to my companion books, starting with U.T.O.P.I.A.

Reactive oxygen species is an older, inaccurate name for electronically modified oxygen derivatives (EMODs), which does not infer or connote radicality, charge or reactivity.

Reactive oxygen species appears to be central to cancer cell apoptosis and electronically modified oxygen derivatives (EMODs) serve as a key tumoricidal agents. This is also true with vitamin D. Thus, I would argue that all of the salutary effects of vitamin D are attributable to its prooxidant activity.

To wit, I have included a few pertinent reference abstracted articles.

Vitamin D is a prooxidant in breast cancer cells

Abstract

The anticancer activity of the hormonal form of vitamin D, 1,25-di-hydroxyvitamin D [1,25(OH)2D], is associated with inhibition of cell cycle progression, induction of differentiation, and apoptosis. In addition, 1,25(OH)2D3 augments the activity of anticancer agents that induce excessive reactive oxygen species generation in their target cells. This study aimed to find out whether 1,25(OH)2D3, acting as a single agent, is a prooxidant in cancer cells. The ratio between oxidized and reduced glulathione and the oxidation-dependent inactivation of glyceraldehyde-3phosphate dehydrogenase (GAPDH) are considered independent markers of cellular reactive oxygen species homeostasis and redox state. Treatment of MCF-7 breast cancer cells with 1,25(OH)2D3 (10-100 nM for 24-48 h) brought about a maximal increase of 41+/-13% (mean +/- SE) in the oxidized/reduced glutathione ratio without affecting total glutathione levels. The in situ activity of glutathione peroxidase and catalase were not affected by 1,25(OH)2D3, as assessed by the rate of H2O2 degradation by MCF-7 cell cultures. Neither did treatment with 1,25(OH)2D3 affect the levels of glutathione reductase or glutathione S-transferase as assayed in cell extracts. The hormone did not affect overall glutathione consumption and efflux as reflected in the rate of decline of total cellular glutathione after inhibition of its synthesis by buthionine sulfoximine. The extent of reversible oxidation-dependent inactivation of GAPDH in situ was determined by comparing the enzyme activity before and after reduction of cell extracts with DTT. The oxidized fraction was 0.13+/-0.02 of total GAPDH in control cultures and increased by 56+/-5.3% after treatment with 1,25(OH)2D3, which did not affect the total reduced enzyme activity. Treatment with 1,25(OH)2D3 resulted in a approximately 40% increase in glucose-6-phosphate dehydrogenase, the rate-limiting enzyme in the generation of NADPH. This enzyme is induced in response to various modes of oxidative challenge in mammalian cells. Taken together, these findings indicate that **1,25(OH)2D3 causes an increase in the overall cellular redox potential that could translate into modulation of redox-sensitive enzymes and transcription factors that regulate cell cycle progression, differentiation, and apoptosis.** (Koren et al, 2001)

The role of ROS in anticancer activity of vitamin D

Abstract

Calcitriol, the hormonal form of vitamin D, enhances the anticancer activity of the immune cytokine tumor necrosis factor, interleukin 1 and interleukin 6 in human breast and renal cell carcinoma cells without affecting the cytotoxic action of interferon-alpha or killer lymphocytes. It also enhances cytotoxicity induced by the anticancer drug doxorubicin, by the redox cycling quinone menadione, and by the reactive oxygen species hydrogen peroxide. The synergistic interaction was accompanied by increased oxidative stress, as manifested by glutathione depletion and was abolished by exposure to the thiol antioxidant N-acetylcysteine. The hormone on its own brought about an increase in the cellular redox state as reflected in the ratio between oxidized and reduced glutathione and glyceraldehyde-3-phosphate dehydrogenase, and a reduction in the expression of the antioxidant enzyme Cu/Zn superoxide dismutase. **These results support the notion that the interplay between active vitamin D derivatives and other anticancer agents such as immune cytokines and anticancer drugs plays a role in the in vivo anticancer activity of vitamin D and that reactive oxygen species are involved in the anticancer activity of vitamin D** on its own and in its cross-talk with other anticancer modalities. (Ravid, Koren, 2003)

Vitamin D(3) and immune cytokines: role of ROS Abstract

It was previously shown that 1,25-dihydroxyvitamin D(3) (1, 25(OH)(2)D(3)) enhances the cytotoxic activity of tumor necrosis factor alpha

(TNFalpha), doxorubicin and menadione. **A feature shared by these anticancer agents is the involvement of reactive oxygen species (ROS) in their action.** In this work we found that 1, 25(OH)(2) D(3) acted synergistically with interleukin 1 beta (IL-1beta) or interleukin 6 (IL-6) to inhibit the proliferation of MCF-7 breast cancer cells. The extent of the synergism was maximal at 1 nM, a concentration at which 1,25(OH)(2)D(3), acting singly, only marginally reduced the cell number. The thiol antioxidant, N-acetylcysteine (NAC) abolished the synergism between IL-1beta or IL-6 and 1,25(OH)(2)D(3), but had only a small protective effect when the cytokines acted alone. **NAC and reduced glutathione (GSH) protected MCF-7 cells from cytotoxicity induced both by TNFalpha alone and by TNFalpha and 1,25(OH)(2)D(3).** A two-day exposure to TNFalpha caused a 27.7+/-3.1% (mean +/- SEM) reduction in GSH content. This effect increased to 46.4+/-5.5% by co-treatment with 1, 25(OH)(2)D(3) which did not affect GSH levels on it own. We conclude that **1,25(OH)(2) D(3) can act synergistically with anticancer cytokines present in the tumor milieu and that ROS plays a mediatory role in this interaction.** (Koren et al, 2000)

Vitamin D(3) enhances ROS chemotherapy of breast cancer cells Abstract

1,25-Dihydroxyvitamin D3 (1,25(OH)2D3), the hormonal form of vitamin D, has anticancer activity in vivo and in vitro. Doxorubicin exerts its cytotoxic effect on tumor cells mainly by two mechanisms: (a) generation of reactive oxygen species (ROS); and (b) inhibition of topoisomerase II. We studied the combined cytotoxic action of 1,25(OH)2D3 and doxorubicin on MCF-7 breast cancer cells. Pretreatement with 1,25(OH)2D3 resulted in enhanced cytotoxicity of doxorubicin. The average enhancing effect after a 72-h pretreatment with 1,25(OH)2D3 (10 nM) followed by a 24-h treatment with 1 microg/ml doxorubicin was 74+/-9% (mean +/- SE). Under these experimental conditions, 1,25(OH)2D3 on its own did not affect cell number or viability. 1,25(OH)2D3 also enhanced the cytotoxic activity of another ROS generating quinone, menadione, but did not affect cytotoxicity induced by the topoisomerase inhibitor etoposide. The antioxidant N-acetylcysteine slightly reduced the cytotoxic activity of doxorubicin but had a marked protective effect against the combined action of 1,25(OH)2D3 and doxorubicin. These results indicate that **ROS are involved in the interaction between 1,25(OH)2D3 and doxorubicin. 1,25(OH)2D3 also increased doxorubicin cytotoxicity in primary cultures of rat cardiomyocytes.** Treatment of MCF-7 cells with 1,25(OH)2D3 alone markedly reduced the activity, protein, and mRNA levels of the cytoplasmic antioxidant enzyme Cu/Zn superoxide dismutase, which indicated that the hormone inhibits its biosynthesis. This reduction in the antioxidant capacity of the cells could account for the synergistic interaction between 1,25(OH)2D3 and doxorubicin and may also suggest increased efficacy of 1,25(OH)2D3 or its analogues in combination with other ROS-generating anticancer therapeutic modalities. (Ravid et al, 1999)

SUMMARIZED NEGATIVE DATA ON VITAMIN D

The Johns Hopkins Bloomberg School of Public Health reminds us that "strong associations" are not proof of causality.

There is a disconnect between the observational studies that have linked low vitamin D to nearly every known health condition and the randomized trials of high-dose vitamin D supplements that have been largely disappointing to date.

"Vitamin D deficiency is quite rare in North Americans at this point in time." (Glenville Jones, a Canadian doctor on the 14-member committee for the US-based Institute of Medicine, 2010) **The only sure benefit of the combination of calcium and vitamin D is bone health. We don't want to base public health recommendations upon a mixed conclusion** where some studies say there is a benefit in cancer and other studies say they don't.

Almost 70% of the U.S. population has insufficient levels of 25(OH)D, when defined as less than 30 ng/mL.

6.6% of whites and 32.3% of blacks had severely low levels of vitamin D in their blood, classified as levels below 15 nanograms per milliliter.

If electing to test vitamin D status, serum 25-hydroxyvitamin D is the accepted biomarker. Although 1,25-OH-D is the active circulating form of vitamin D, measuring this level is not helpful because it is quickly and tightly regulated by the kidney. True deficiency would be evident only by measuring 25-OH-D. Of note, questions have been raised regarding the need for standardization of assays. (Binkley et al, 2004)

A large laboratory (Quest Diagnostics) recently reported the possibility of thousands of incorrect vitamin D level results. (Pollack, 2009)

The **U.S. National Cancer Institute** noted that its studies conducted on the effects of vitamin D on cancer may not be completely accurate because studying a person's blood vitamin level at a single point in time, as many studies do, may not give an accurate picture of his or her true levels. Moreover, many studies don't use high enough doses to see the benefits.

Controversy exists regarding the optimum level of serum 25-hydroxyvitamin D in a healthy population. Most experts agree that serum vitamin D levels <20 ng/mL represent deficiency. However, some experts recommend aiming for a higher minimum target level of 30 ng/mL of 25-hydroxyvitamin D in a healthy population. **Vitamin D intoxication can occur when serum levels are greater than 150 ng/mL.**

Observational studies suggest that shooting for blood levels above 50 ng/mL may be associated with an increased risk of pancreatic cancer, cardiovascular disease and an increased risk of death.

More than 2,000 IU a day can cause toxicity problems including excessive urination, high blood pressure, nausea, weight loss, fatigue, calcium deposits in soft tissues (kidney stones) and kidney damage.

It is hard to consume 600 IUs of vitamin D from food alone.

Massive doses of 10,000 IU daily or more can put you at risk of developing high calcium levels in the blood, or in the urine, which could cause calcification of blood vessels, kidney problems and kidney stones, especially if calcium intake is also high.

Steroid drugs like prednisone, weight loss drugs like orlistat (Alli) and the cholesterol-lowering drug cholestyramine (Questran) can reduce the absorption of vitamin D.

A National Cancer Institute study was the latest to report no cancer protection from vitamin D and the possibility of an increased risk of pancreatic cancer in people with the very highest D levels.

Even though the vitamin has been associated with 137 outcomes in reports (including skeletal, malignant, cardiovascular,

autoimmune, infectious, metabolic and other diseases), the researchers found only 10 had been well studied. The only evidence of benefit appeared to be for birth weight and the mother's vitamin D status; there were "probable" associations with a few other outcomes -- dental caries in children, maternal vitamin D levels at term, and parathyroid hormone levels in dialysis patients -- but better-designed trials are needed to draw firmer conclusions. The findings cast doubt on vitamin D for osteoporosis, and it "might not be as essential as previously thought in maintaining bone mineral density. (Quoted by K. Fiore, 2014 in MedPage Today referring to an umbrella review of 268 observational studies and meta-analyses published in BMJ)

In a review of seven trials totaling nearly 3,200 patients, the vitamin had no significant effect on depressive symptoms overall, Jonathan Shaffer, PhD, of Columbia University Medical Center, in New York City, and colleagues reported in *Psychosomatic Medicine*. However, when looking specifically at patients who had clinically significant depressive symptoms or depressive disorder, the researchers found that there did appear to be a moderately significant effect of vitamin D supplementation on symptoms.

Supplementation with 1000 IU/day vitamin D_3 did not significantly reduce the incidence or duration of URTI (upper respiratory tract infections) in adults with a baseline serum 25-hydroxyvitamin D level $\geq$12 ng/mL. Vitamin D and calcium, whatever their other benefits may be, have no effect on upper respiratory tract infections. (Rees et al, 2013)

Simply supplementing vitamin D as part of a dietary intervention won't necessarily aid weight loss, unless patients actually achieve levels of 25 (OH)D of 32 ng/mL or more. (Mason et al, 2014)

Vitamin D_3 did not reduce the rate of first treatment failure or exacerbation in adults with persistent asthma and vitamin D insufficiency. These findings do not support a strategy of therapeutic vitamin D_3 supplementation in patients with symptomatic asthma. (Castro et al, VIDA Trial, 2014)

There was also no significant reduction in the secondary end points related to asthma control, airway function, quality of life, or airway inflammation. (Castro et al, VIDA Trial, 2014)

Levels of 25(OH)D are all over the map, varying considerably by country, sex, and time of year.

More than 2,000 IU a day can cause toxicity problems including excessive urination, high blood pressure, nausea, weight loss, fatigue, calcium deposits in soft tissues (kidney stones) and kidney damage.

Observational studies suggest that shooting for blood levels above 50 ng/mL may be associated with an increased risk of pancreatic cancer, cardiovascular disease and an increased risk of death.

Massive doses of 10,000 IU daily or more can put you at risk of developing high calcium levels in the blood, or in the urine, which could cause calcification of blood vessels, kidney problems and kidney stones, especially if calcium intake is also high.

Even though the vitamin has been associated with 137 outcomes in reports (including skeletal, malignant, cardiovascular, autoimmune, infectious, metabolic and other diseases), the researchers found only 10 had been well studied.

The only evidence of benefit appeared to be for birth weight and the mother's vitamin D status; there were "probable" associations with a few other outcomes -- dental caries in children, maternal vitamin D levels at term, and parathyroid hormone levels in dialysis patients -- but better-designed trials are needed to draw firmer conclusions.

In a review of seven trials totaling nearly 3,200 patients, the vitamin had no significant effect on depressive symptoms overall.

Vitamin D and calcium, whatever their other benefits may be, have no effect on upper respiratory tract infections.

Vitamin D_3 did not reduce the rate of first treatment failure or exacerbation in adults with persistent asthma and vitamin D insufficiency. There was also no significant reduction in the secondary end points related to asthma control, airway function, quality of life, or airway inflammation.

The only sure benefit of the combination of calcium and vitamin D is bone health.

Evidence does not support the argument that vitamin D only supplementation increases bone mineral density or reduces the risk of fractures or falls in older people. Vitamin D alone is unlikely to prevent fracture. Overall there is a small but significant increase in gastrointestinal symptoms and renal disease associated with vitamin D or its analogues. Calcitriol is associated with an increased incidence of hypercalcaemia. (Avenell et al, 2009)

Highly convincing evidence of a clear role of vitamin D with highly significant results in both randomized and observational evidence does not exist for any outcome, but associations with a selection of outcomes are probable.

Suggestive evidence exists that high vitamin D concentrations are linked to an increased rate of falls and risk of hypercalcaemia in chronic kidney disease patients not requiring dialysis.

No universal consensus exists on the optimal vitamin D intake or the optimal plasma concentrations of 25-hydroxyvitamin D.

A very recent meta-analysis of randomized controlled trials on bone mineral density failed to show a definite association and concluded that widespread use of vitamin D supplementation for prevention of osteoporosis is not supported by the evidence.

Two recent Cochrane reviews failed to find a protective effect of vitamin D only supplementation on the risk or rate of falling in older adults.

Randomized controlled trials of vitamin D for autoimmune and cancer related outcomes are clearly lacking.

Vitamin D is more likely to be a correlate marker of overall health and not causally involved in disease.

There is an absence of meta-analyses in relation to autoimmune disease and the absence of meta-analyses of randomized clinical trials of vitamin D supplementation in respect of cancer, cognitive, and infectious disease outcomes.

High 25(OH)D concentrations were not associated with a lower risk of cancer, except colorectal cancer. However, results from intervention studies did not show an effect of vitamin D

Prof Randolph M. Howes MD,PhD

supplementation on disease occurrence, including colorectal cancer.

Continuing widespread use of vitamin D for osteoporosis prevention in community-dwelling adults without specific risk factors for vitamin D deficiency seems to be inappropriate.

There is little reason to prescribe vitamin D supplements to healthy adults to reduce the risk of diseases or fractures, say researchers writing in the Lancet. They found no significant reduction in risk in any area after analyzing more than 100 trials.

They found that vitamin D supplementation does not change the relative risk of heart disease, stroke or cerebrovascular disease, cancer and fractures by a noticeable amount, equivalent to 15%.

People with low vitamin D levels are at increased risk of dying from cancer — but only if they have already had cancer.

The study said there was also "uncertainty as to whether vitamin D with or without calcium reduces the risk of death".

The New Zealand researchers concluded: **In view of our findings, there is little justification for prescribing vitamin D supplements to prevent myocardial infarction or ischemic heart disease, stroke or cerebrovascular disease, cancer, or fractures, or to reduce the risk of death in unselected community-dwelling individuals. Investigators and funding bodies should consider the probable futility of undertaking similar trials of vitamin D to investigate any of these endpoints.** (Bolland et al, 2014)

However, very recently, Northwestern University researchers said that vitamin D can help reduce the risk of aggressive prostate cancer in men.

Vitamin D supplements did not reduce hip fracture risk by more than 15% in hospital patients and, when given with calcium, did not lessen the risk in healthy individuals either.

Another study found no concrete evidence to suggest that vitamin D supplements are effective in preventing accidental falls in older people.

Vitamin D, Umbrella review, 2014

On the basis of the available evidence, **an association between vitamin D concentrations and birth weight, dental caries in children, maternal vitamin D concentrations at term, and parathyroid hormone concentrations in patients with chronic kidney disease requiring dialysis is probable.** (Vitamin D, Umbrella review, 2014)

Evidence does not support the argument that vitamin D only supplementation increases bone mineral density or reduces the risk of fractures or falls in older people. (Vitamin D, Umbrella review, 2014)

Highly convincing evidence of a clear role of vitamin D does not exist for any outcome, but associations with a selection of outcomes are probable. (Vitamin D, Umbrella review, 2014)

The composite literature is often confusing and has led to heated debates about the optimal concentrations of vitamin D and related guidelines for supplementation. (Vitamin D, Umbrella review, 2014)

For only six (8%) of the 76 unique outcomes, the systematic reviews concluded that a definite association existed. These were rheumatoid arthritis activity, colorectal cancer, hypertension in children, bacterial vaginosis in pregnant women, falls in older people, and rickets in children; for all these outcomes, higher concentrations of vitamin D were associated with lower risk. (Vitamin D, Umbrella review, 2014)

Overall, 13 (23%) of the 57 meta-analyses of randomized controlled trials reported a nominally statistically significant summary result, and these were related to the following outcomes: total cholesterol concentrations, birth weight, head circumference at birth, maternal vitamin D concentrations at term, balance sway, femoral neck bone mineral density, muscle strength, non-vertebral fractures, rate of falls, dental caries in children, parathyroid hormone concentrations in patients with chronic kidney disease (requiring or not requiring dialysis), and risk of hypercalcaemia in patients with chronic kidney disease not requiring dialysis. (Vitamin D, Umbrella review, 2014)

Highly convincing evidence of a clear role of vitamin D with highly significant results in both randomized and observational evidence does not exist <u>for any outcome.</u> (Vitamin D, Umbrella review, 2014)

On the other hand, <u>suggestive evidence exists that high vitamin D concentrations are linked to an increased rate of falls and risk of hypercalcaemia in chronic kidney disease patients not requiring dialysis.</u> (Vitamin D, Umbrella review, 2014)

<u>No universal consensus exists on the optimal vitamin D intake or the optimal plasma concentrations of 25-hydroxyvitamin D.</u> (Vitamin D, Umbrella review, 2014)

****

A very recent meta-analysis of randomized controlled trials on bone mineral density failed to show a definite association and **<u>concluded that widespread use of vitamin D supplementation for prevention of osteoporosis is not supported by the evidence</u>, a fact that is also verified by the findings of our review.** (Reid et al, 2014)

Two recent Cochrane reviews failing to find a protective effect of vitamin D only supplementation on the risk or rate of falling in older adults (both in care facilities or hospitals and in the community). (Cameron et al, 2012)

In conclusion, although vitamin D has been extensively studied in relation to a range of outcomes and some indications exist that low plasma vitamin D concentrations might be linked to several diseases, **firm universal conclusions about its benefits cannot be drawn. Randomized controlled trials of vitamin D for autoimmune and cancer related outcomes are clearly lacking**. (Vitamin D, Umbrella review, 2014)

Vitamin D is more likely to be a correlate marker of overall health and not causally involved in disease. (Vitamin D, Umbrella review, 2014)

This review highlights the absence of meta-analyses in relation to autoimmune disease and the absence of meta-analyses of randomized clinical trials of vitamin D supplementation in respect of cancer, cognitive, and infectious disease outcomes. (Vitamin D, Umbrella review, 2014)

High 25(OH)D concentrations were not associated with a lower risk of cancer, except colorectal cancer. (Autier et al, 2014) But, results from <u>intervention studies</u> **did not show an effect of vitamin D supplementation on disease occurrence, including colorectal cancer.**

The discrepancy between observational and intervention studies <u>**suggests**</u> that **low 25(OH)D is a marker of ill health.** (Autier et al, 2014)

Findings from **recent meta-analyses of vitamin D supplementation without co-administration of calcium have not shown fracture prevention.** (Reid et al, 2014) **Results of our meta-analysis showed a small benefit at the femoral neck with heterogeneity among trials. No effect at any other site was reported, including the total hip.**

Continuing widespread use of vitamin D for osteoporosis prevention in community-dwelling adults without specific risk factors for vitamin D deficiency seems to be inappropriate. (Reid et al, 2014)

<u>**In view of our findings, there is little justification for prescribing vitamin D supplements to prevent myocardial infarction or ischemic heart disease, stroke or cerebrovascular disease, cancer, or fractures, or to reduce the risk of death in unselected community-dwelling individuals. Investigators and funding bodies should consider the probable futility of undertaking similar trials of vitamin D to investigate any of these endpoints.**</u> (Bolland et al, 2014)

<u>**There is little reason to prescribe vitamin D supplements to healthy adults to reduce the risk of diseases or fractures**</u>, say researchers writing in the Lancet. **They found no significant reduction in risk in any area after analyzing more than 100 trials.** (Bolland et al, 2014)

<u>**Vitamin D alone is unlikely to prevent fracture.**</u> **Overall there is a small but significant increase in gastrointestinal symptoms and renal disease associated with vitamin D or its analogues. Calcitriol is associated with an increased incidence of hypercalcaemia.** (Avenell et al, 2009)

A large number of the <u>observational studies</u> suggested that there were benefits from high vitamin D - that it could reduce

the risk of cardiovascular events by up to 58%, diabetes by up to 38% and colorectal cancer by up to 33%. But the results of the clinical trials - where participants were given vitamin D supplements - <u>found no reduction in risk</u>, even in people who started out with low vitamin D levels. (Autier et al, 2014)

CONCLUSION

Now, you have seen the relevant data. Is vitamin D a "miracle" or a "myth"?

As you may conclude, earlier studies indicated that vitamin D was rather miraculous but more reliable recent studies have debunked many of the hyperbolic claims made by those marketing this product to an uninformed public. In addition, many of the unreliable conclusions have been used to convince physicians of the unjustified benefits of supplemental vitamin D.

Still, we must respect the fact that certain levels of vitamin D are, indeed, necessary for healthful living. Choose wisely when purchasing unproven supplements for you and your loved ones. And please remember that "more" is not necessarily better.

References

(Adorini, Penna, 2008) (Adorini L, Penna G. Control of autoimmune diseases by the vitamin D endocrine system. *Nat Clin Pract Rheumatol* 2008; 4: 404–12)

(Afzal et al, 2013) (Afzal S, Bojesen SE, Nordestgaard BG. Low 25-hydroxyvitamin D and risk of type 2 diabetes: a prospective cohort study and metaanalysis. Clin Chem. 2013;59:381–91)

(Al-Aly, 2007) (Al-Aly Z. Vitamin D as a novel nontraditional risk factor for mortality in hemodialysis patients: the need for randomized trials. *Kidney Int* 2007;72: 909–11)

(Anderson et al, 2010) (Anderson JL, May HT, Horne BD, Bair TL, Hall NL, Carlquist JF, Lappé DL, Muhlestein JB, Intermountain Heart Collaborative (IHC) Study Group Relation of vitamin D deficiency to cardiovascular risk factors, disease status, and incident events in a general healthcare population. Am J Cardiol. 2010;106:963–8)

(Autier et al, 2014) (Autier P, Boniol M, Pizot C, Mullie P. Vitamin D status and ill health: a systematic review. Lancet Diabetes Endocrinol. 2014;2:76-89)

(Autier, Gandini, 2007) (Autier P, Gandini S. Vitamin D supplementation and total mortality. *Arch Intern Med* 2007; 167: 1730–7)

(Avenell et al, 2005) (Avenell A, Gillespie WJ, O'Connell DC. Vitamin D and vitamin D analogues for preventing fractures associated with involutional and postmenopausal osteoporosis. *Cochrane Database Syst Rev* 2005; (3):CD000227)

(Avenell et al, 2009) (Avenell A, Gillespie WJ, Gillespie LD, O'Connell D. Vitamin D and vitamin D analogues for preventing fractures associated with involutional and post-menopausal osteoporosis. Cochrane Database Syst Rev. 2009;(2):CD000227)

(Bailey et al, 2010) (Bailey RL, Dodd KW, Goldman JA, Gahche JJ, Dwyer JT, Moshfegh AJ, et al. Estimation of total usual calcium and vitamin D intakes in the United States. J Nutr. 2010;140:817-22)

(Bergman et al, 2013) (Bergman P, Lindh AU, Björkhem-Bergman L, Lindh JD. Vitamin D and respiratory tract infections: A systematic review and meta-analysis of randomized controlled trials. PLoS One. 2013;8:e65835)

(Bilinski, Boyages, 2013) (Bilinski K, Boyages S. Evidence of overtesting for vitamin D in Australia: an analysis of 4.5 years of Medicare Benefits Schedule (MBS) data. BMJ Open. 2013 Jun 20;3(6). pii: e002955. doi: 10.1136/bmjopen-2013-002955)

(Binkley et al, 2004) (Binkley N, Krueger D, Cowgill CS, et al. Assay variation confounds the diagnosis of hypovitaminosis D: a call for standardization. *J Clin Endocrinol Metab* 2004; 89: 3152–7)

(Bischoff_Ferrari et al, 2004) (Bischoff-Ferrari HA, Dawson-Hughes B, Willett WC, et al. Effect of vitamin D on falls: a meta-analysis. *JAMA* 2004; 291: 1999–2006)

(Bischoff-Ferrari et al, 2005) (Bischoff-Ferrari HA, Willett WC, Wong JB, Giovannucci E, Dietrich T, Dawson-Hughes B. Fracture prevention with vitamin D supplementation: a meta-analysis of randomized controlled trials. JAMA. 2005;293:2257-64)

(Bischoff-Ferrari et al, 2009) (Bischoff-Ferrari HA, Willett WC, Wong JB, et al. Prevention of nonvertebral fractures with oral vitamin D dose dependency. A meta-analysis of randomized controlled trials. *Arch Intern Med* 2009; 169:551–61)

(Bischoff-Ferrari et al, 2009a) (Bischoff-Ferrari HA, Dawson-Hughes B, Staehelin HB, Orav JE, Stuck AE, Theiler R, Wong JB, Egli A, Kiel DP, Henschkowski J. Fall prevention with supplemental and active forms of vitamin D: a meta-analysis of randomised controlled trials. BMJ. 2009a;339:b3692. doi: 10.1136/bmj.b3692)

(Bischoff-Ferrari, et al 2012) (Bischoff-Ferrari HA, Willett WC, Orav EJ, Lips P, Meunier PJ, Lyons RA, et al. A pooled analysis of vitamin D dose requirements for fracture prevention [correction in N Engl J Med 2012;367:481]. N Engl J Med. 2012;367:40-9)

(Bolland et al, 2014) (Bolland MJ et al. The effect of vitamin D supplementation on skeletal, vascular, or cancer outcomes: a trial sequential meta-analysis. The Lancet Diabetes & Endocrinology, Vol 2, Issue 4, Pages 307-320)

(Bonnen et al, 2007) (Boonen S, Lips P, Bouillon R, Bischoff-Ferrari HA, Vanderschueren D, Haetiens P. Need for additional calcium to reduce the risk of hip fracture with vitamin D supplementation: evidence from a comparative meta-analysis of randomized controlled trials. *J Clin Endocrinol Metab*2007; 92: 1415–23)

(Broe et al, 2007) (Broe KE, Chen TC, Weinberg J, et al. A higher dose of vitamin D reduces the risk of falls in nursing home residents: a randomized multiple-dose study. *J Am Geriatr Soc* 2007; 55: 234–9)

(Buell et al, 2008) (Buell JS, Dawson-Hughes B. Vitamin D and neuro-cognitive dysfunction: preventing "D"ecline? *Mol Aspects Med* 2008; 29: 415–22)

(Cantorna, 2006) (Vitamin D and its role in immunology: multiple sclerosis, and inflammatory bowel disease. Cantorna MT. Prog Biophys Mol Biol. 2006 Sep;92(1):60-4)

(Cameron et al, 2012) (Cameron ID, Gillespie LD, Robertson MC, Murray GR, Hill KD, Cumming RG, et al. Interventions for preventing falls in older people in care facilities and hospitals. Cochrane Database Syst Rev. 2012;(12):CD005465)

(Castro et al, VIDA Trial, 2014) (Effect of Vitamin D_3 on Asthma Treatment Failures in Adults With Symptomatic Asthma and Lower Vitamin D Levels. The VIDA Randomized Clinical Trial. Mario Castro. May 28, 2014, Vol 311, No. 20. pp 2083-2091)

(Choi et al, 2014) (Choi YM, Kim WG, Kim TY, Bae SJ, Kim HK, Jang EK, Jeon MJ, Han JM, Lee SH, Baek JH, Shong YK, Kim WB. Low levels of serum vitamin D3 are associated with autoimmune thyroid disease in pre-menopausal women. Thyroid. 2014 Apr;24(4):655-61)

(Churilla et al, 2012) (Churilla TM, Brereton HD, Klem M, Peters CA. Vitamin D deficiency is widespread in cancer patients and correlates with advanced stage disease: a community oncology experience. Nutr Cancer. 2012;64:521–5)

(Coussens et al, 2012) (Coussens A.K. Wilkinson R.J. Hanifa Y. Nikolayevskyy V. Elkington P.T. Islam K. Timms P.M. Venton T.R. Bothamley G.H. Packe G.E. Darmalingam M. Davidson R.N. Milburn H.J. Baker L.V. Barker R.D. Mein C.A. Bhaw-Rosun L. Nuamah R. Young D.B. Drobniewski F.A. Griffiths C.J. Martineau A.R. (2012) Vitamin D accelerates resolution of inflammatory responses during tuberculosis treatment, Proc Natl Acad Sci U S A, 109(38),15449-15454)

(Cranney et al, 2008) (Cranney A, Weiler HA, O'Donnell S, Puil L. Summary of evidence-based review on vitamin D efficacy and safety in relation to bone health. Am J Clin Nutr 2008; 88(Suppl): 513S–9S)

(Dobnig et al, 2008) (Dobnig H, Pilz S, Scharnagl H, et al. Independent association of low serum 25-hydroxyvitamin D and 1,25-dihydroxyvita-min D levels with all-cause and cardiovascular mortality. Arch Intern Med 2008; 168:1340–9)

(Effraimidis et al, 2012) (Effraimidis G, Badenhoop K, Tijssen JG, Wiersinga WM. Eur J Endocrinol. 2012 Jul;167(1):43-8. doi: 10.1530/EJE-12-0048. Epub 2012 Apr 19)

(Freedman et al, 2007) (Freedman DM, Looker AC, Chang SC, Graubard BI. Prospective study of serum vitamin D and cancer mortality in the United States. J Natl Cancer Inst 2007; 99: 1594–602)

(FSA, 2012) (Food Standards Agency, National Diet and Nutrition Survey Headline results from Years 1, 2 and 3 (combined) of the rolling program (2008/2009 – 2010/11 https://www.gov.uk/government/publications/national-diet-and-nutrition-survey-results-from-years 1-to-4-combined-of-the-rolling-programme-for-2008-and-2009-to-2011-and-2012 Last accessed June 2014)

(Gagnon et al, 2012) (Gagnon C, Lu ZX, Magliano DJ, Dunstan DW, Shaw JE, Zimmet PZ, Sikaris K, Ebeling PR, Daly RM. Low serum 25-hydroxyvitamin D is associated with increased risk of the development of the metabolic syndrome at five years: results from a national, population-based prospective study (The Australian Diabetes, Obesity and Lifestyle Study: AusDiab) J Clin Endocrinol Metab. 2012;97:1953–61)

(Gallagher et al, 2012) (Gallagher JC, Sai A, Templin T 2nd, Smith L. Dose response to vitamin D supplementation in postmenopausal women: a randomized trial. Ann Intern Med. 2012 Mar 20;156(6):425-37)

(Gandini et al, 2011) (Gandini S, Boniol M, Haukka J, Byrnes G, Cox B, Sneyd MJ, Mullie P, Autier P. Meta-analysis of observational studies of serum 25-hydroxyvitamin D levels and colorectal, breast and prostate cancer and colorectal adenoma. Int J Cancer. 2011;128(6):1414-24.)

(Garland et al, 2006) (Garland CF, Garland FC, Gorham ED, et al. The role of vitamin D in cancer prevention. Am J Public Health 2006; 96: 252–61)

(Garland et al, 2014) (Cedric F. Garland, June Jiwon Kim, Sharif Burgette Mohr, Edward Doerr Gorham, William B. Grant, Edward L. Giovannucci, Leo Baggerly, Heather Hofflich, Joe Wesley Ramsdell, Kenneth Zeng, Robert P. Heaney. Meta-analysis of All-Cause Mortality According to Serum 25-Hydroxyvitamin D. American Journal of Public Health, 2014; e1 DOI: 10.2105/AJPH.2014.302034)

(Gillespie et al, 2012) (Gillespie LD, Robertson MC, Gillespie WJ, Sherrington C, Gates S, Clemson LM, et al. Interventions for preventing falls in older people living in the community. Cochrane Database Syst Rev. 2012;(9):CD007146)

(Giovannucci et al, 2006) (Giovannucci E, Liu Y, Rimm EB, et al. Prospective study of predictors of vitamin D statius and cancer incidence and mortality in men. J Natl Cancer Inst 2006; 98: 451–9)

(Grant, 2002) (Grant WB. An estimate of premature cancer mortality in the U.S. due to inadequate doses of solar ultraviolet-B radiation. Cancer. 2002;94:1867–75)

(Grant, 2010) (Grant WB. The prevalence of multiple sclerosis in 3 US communities: the role of vitamin D. Prev Chronic Dis.2010;7:A89–, author reply A90)

(Grant, 2012) (Grant WB. Ecological studies of the UVB-vitamin D-cancer hypothesis. Anticancer Res. 2012;32:223–36)

(Grober et al, 2013) (Gröber U, Spitz J, Reichrath J, Kisters K, Holick MF. Vitamin D: Update 2013: From rickets prophylaxis to general preventive healthcare. Dermatoendocrinol. 2013 Jun 1;5(3):331-47. doi: 10.4161/derm.26738. Epub 2013 Nov 5)

(Harandi et al, 2014) (Vitamin D and multiple sclerosis. Harandi AA, Harandi AA, Pakdaman H, Sahraian MA. Iran J Neurol. 2014;13(1):1-6)

(Health Quality Ontario, 2010) (Clinical utility of vitamin d testing: an evidence-based analysis. Ont Health Technol Assess Ser. 2010;10(2):1-93. Epub 2010 Feb 1)

(Hickey, Roberts, 2013) (Hickey S. Roberts H. (2013) Vitamin C and cancer: is there a role for oral vitamin C? JOM, 28(1), 33-46)

(Ho et al, 2012) (Ho SL, Alappat L, Awad AB. Vitamin D and multiple sclerosis. Crit Rev Food Sci Nutr. 2012;52:980–7)

(Hobday, 1997) (Hobday R.A. (1997) Sunlight therapy and solar architecture, Med Hist, 41(4), 455-472)

(Holick, 2004) (Holick MF. Sunlight and vitamin D for bone health and prevention of autoimmune diseases, cancers, and cardiovascular disease. Am J Clin Nutr 2004; 80(6 Suppl): 1678S–88S)

(Holick, 2010) (Holick MF. Vitamin D and Health: Evolution, Biologic Functions, and Recommended Dietary Intakes of Vitamin D. In Vitamin D: Physiology, Molecular Biology and Clinical Applications by Holick MF. Humana Press, 2010)

(Hollick et al, 2012) (Holick MF, Binkley NC, Bischoff-Ferrari HA, Gordon CM, Hanley DA, Heaney RP, Murad MH, Weaver CM. Guidelines for preventing and treating vitamin D deficiency and insufficiency revisited. J Clin Endocrinol Metab.2012;97:1153–8)

(Howes, 2012) (Antioxidant Links To Deadly Unintended Consequences. Prof. R.M. Howes, MD, PhD. CreateSpace and Free Radical Publishing Co, USA, © 2012)

(Hujoel, 2013) (Hujoel PP.Vitamin D and dental caries in controlled clinical trials: systematic review and meta-analysis. Nutr Rev.2013;71:88–97)

(Inaquma et al, 2008) (Inaguma D, Nagaya H, Hara K, et al. Relationship between serum 1,25-dihydroxyvitamin D and mortality in patients with pre-dialysis chronic kidney disease. Clin Exp Nephrol 2008; 12: 126–31)

(Jackson et al, 2006) (Jackson RD, LaCroix AZ, Gass M, et al; Women's Health Initiative Investigators. Calcium plus vitamin D supplementation and the risk of fractures. N Engl J Med. 2006;354:669-683)

(Javanbakht et al, 2010) (Javanbakht M, Keshavarz S, Mirshafiey A, Djalali M, Siassi F, Eshraghian M, Firooz A, Seirafi H, Ehsani A, Chamari M. The effects of vitamins e and d supplementation on erythrocyte superoxide dismutase and catalase in atopic dermatitis. Iran J Public Health. 2010;39(1):57-63. Epub 2010 Mar 31)

(Koh et al, 2012) (Koh G.C. Hawthorne G. Turner A.M. Kunst H. Dedicoat M. (2012) Tuberculosis incidence correlates with sunshine: an ecological 28-year time series study, PLoS One, 8(3), e57752)

(Koren et al, 2001) (Koren R, Hadari-Naor I, Zuck E, Rotem C, Liberman UA, Ravid A. Vitamin D is a prooxidant in breast cancer cells. Cancer Res. 2001 Feb 15;61(4):1439-44)

(Koren et al, 2000) (Koren R, Rocker D, Kotestiano O, Liberman UA, Ravid A. Synergistic anticancer activity of 1,25-dihydroxyvitamin D(3) and immune cytokines: the involvement of reactive oxygen species. J Steroid Biochem Mol Biol. 2000 Jun;73(3-4):105-12)

(Knight et al, 2007) (Knight JA, Lesosky M, Barnett H, Raboud JM, Vieth R. Vitamin D and reduced risk of breast cancer: a population-based case-control study. Cancer Epidemiol Biomarkers Prev. 2007;16:422–9)

(Kragt et al, 2009) (Kragt JJ, van Amerongen BM, Killestein J, et al. Higher levels of 25-hydroxyvitamin D are associated with a lower incidence of multiple sclerosis only in women. Mult Scler 2009; 15: 9–15)

(Kulie et al, 2009) (Vitamin D: An Evidence-Based Review. Teresa Kulie et al, J Am Board Fam Med. November-December 2009 vol. 22 no. 6 698-706)

(Lappe et al, 2007) (Lappe JM, Travers-Gustafson D, Davies KM, Recker RR, Heaney RP. Vitamin D and calcium supplementation reduces cancer risk: results of a randomized trial. Am J Clin Nutr 2007; 85: 1586–91)

(Liu et al, 2007) (Liu P.T. Stenger S. Tang D.H. Modlin R.L. (2007) Cutting edge: vitamin D-mediated human antimicrobial activity against Mycobacterium tuberculosis is dependent on the induction of cathelicidin, J Immunol, 179(4), 2060-2063)

(Lowdon, 2011) (Lowdon J. Rickets: concerns over the worldwide increase. Journal of Family Healthcare. 2011;21(2):25-9)

(Luscombe et al, 2001) (Luscombe CJ, Fryer AA, French ME, Liu S, Saxby MF, Jones PW, Strange RC. Exposure to ultraviolet radiation: association with susceptibility and age at presentation with prostate cancer. Lancet. 2001;358:641–2)

(Mason et al, 2014) (Mason C et al. Vitamin D3 supplementation during weight loss: a double-blind randomized controlled trial. Am J Clin Nutr May 2014 Vol. 99. no 5. 1015- 1025)

(Mohr et al, 2008) (Mohr SB, Garland CF, Gorham ED, Garland FC. The association between ultraviolet B irradiance, vitamin D status and incidence rates of type 1 diabetes in 51 regions worldwide. Diabetologia. 2008;51:1391–8. doi: 10.1007/s00125-008-1061-5)

(Munger et al, 2004) (Munger KL, Zhang S.M, O'Reilly E, et al. Vitamin D intake and incidence of multiple sclerosis. *Neurology* 2004; 62: 60–5)

(NOS, 2013) (National Osteoporosis Society. 2013. Vitamin D and Bone Health: A Practical Clinical Guideline for Patient Management. http://www.nos.org.uk/document.doc?id=1352 Last accessed June 2014)

(Oudshoom et al, 2008) (Oudshoorn C, Mattace-Raso FU, van der Velde N, Colin EM, van der Cammen TJ. Higher serum vitamin D3 levels are associated with better cognitive test performance in patients with Alzheimer's disease. *Dement Geriatr Cogn Disord* 2008; 25: 539–43)

(Pellar, Stephensen, 1937) (Peller S, Stephenson CS. Skin Irritation and Cancer in the US Navy. Am J Med Sci. 1937;194:326–33)

(Pittas et al, 2007) (Pittas AG, Lau J, Hu FB, Dawson-Hughes B. The role of vitamin D and calcium in type 2 diabetes. A systematic review and meta-analysis. *J Clin Endocrinol Metab* 2007; 92: 2017–29)

(Plum et al, 2010) (Plum LA and Deluca HF. The Functional Metabolism and Molecular Biology of Vitamin D Action. In Vitamin D: Physiology, Molecular Biology and Clinical Applications by Holick MF. Humana Press, 2010)

(Pollack, 2009) (Pollack A. *Quest acknowledges errors in vitamin D tests.* Available at:http://www.nytimes.com/2009/01/08/business/08labtest. html. Accessed 17 September 2009)

(Prentice et al, 2013) (Prentice RL, Pettinger MB, Jackson RD, et al. Health risks and benefits from calcium and vitamin D supplementation: Women's Health Initiative clinical trial and cohort study. Osteoporos Int. 2013;24:567-580)

(Prince et al, 2008) (Prince RL, Adustin N, Devine A, et al. Effects of ergocalciferol added to calcium on the risk of falls in elderly high-risk women. *Arch Intern Med* 2008; 168: 103–8)

(Ravid et al, 1999) (Ravid A, Rocker D, Machlenkin A, Rotem C, Hochman A, Kessler-Ickekson G, Liberman UA, Koren R. 1,25-Dihydroxyvitamin D3 enhances the susceptibility of breast cancer cells to doxorubicin-induced oxidative damage. Cancer Res. 1999 Feb 15;59(4):862-7)

(Ravid, Koren, 2003) (Ravid A, Koren R. The role of reactive oxygen species in the anticancer activity of vitamin D. Recent Results Cancer Res. 2003;164:357-67)

(Rees et al, 2013) (Rees J et al, Vitamin D3 supplementation and upper respiratory tract infections in a randomized controlled trial. Clin Infect Dis. (2013) 57 (10): 1384-1392)

(Reid et al, 2014) (Reid IR, Bolland MJ, Grey A. Effects of vitamin D supplements on bone mineral density: a systematic review and meta-analysis. Lancet. 2014;383:146-55)

(Rizzoli et al, 2013) (Rizzoli R, Boonen S, Brandi ML, Bruyère O, Cooper C, Kanis JA, Kaufman JM, Ringe JD, Weryha G, Reginster JY. Vitamin D supplementation in elderly or postmenopausal women: a 2013 update of the 2008 recommendations from the European Society for Clinical and Economic Aspects of Osteoporosis and Osteoarthritis (ESCEO). Curr Med Res Opin. 2013 Apr;29(4):305-13)

(Ross et al, 2011) (Ross AC, Manson JE, Abrams SA, Aloia JF, Brannon PM, Clinton SK, et al. The 2011 report on dietary reference intakes for calcium and vitamin D from the Institute of Medicine: what clinicians need to know. J Clin Endocrinol Metab. 2011;96:53-8)

(Santini et al, 2010) (Santini D, Galluzzo S, Vincenzi B, Zoccoli A, Ferraro E, Lippi C, Altomare V, Tonini G, Bertoldo F. Longitudinal evaluation of vitamin D plasma levels during anthracycline- and docetaxel-based adjuvant chemotherapy in early-stage breast cancer patients. Ann Oncol. 2010;21:185-6)

(Schottker et al, 2013) (Schöttker B, Haug U, Schomburg L, Köhrle J, Perna L, Müller H, Holleczek B, Brenner H. Strong associations of 25-hydroxyvitamin D concentrations with all-cause, cardiovascular, cancer, and respiratory disease mortality in a large cohort study. Am J Clin Nutr. 2013;97:782-93)

(Shin et al, 2014) (Low serum vitamin D is associated with anti-thyroid peroxidase antibody in autoimmune thyroiditis. Shin DY, Kim KJ, Kim D, Hwang S, Lee EJ. Yonsei Med J. 2014 Mar;55(2):476-81)

(Smolders et al, 2008) (Smolders J, Damoiseaux J, Menheere P, Hupperts R. Vitamin D as an immune modulator in multiple sclerosis, a review. *J Neuroimmunol* 2008;194: 7–17)

(Sohl et al, 2013) (Sohl E, van Schoor NM, de Jongh RT, Visser M, Deeg DJ, Lips P. Vitamin D status is associated with functional limitations and functional decline in older individuals. J Clin Endocrinol Metab. 2013;98:E1483–90. doi: 10.1210/jc.2013-1698)

(Sorensen et al, 2012) (Sørensen IM, Joner G, Jenum PA, Eskild A, Torjesen PA, Stene LC. Maternal serum levels of 25-hydroxy-vitamin D during pregnancy and risk of type 1 diabetes in the offspring. Diabetes. 2012;61:175–8)

(Steingrimsdottir et al, 2014) (Hip fractures and bone mineral density in the elderly--importance of serum 25-hydroxyvitamin D. Steingrimsdottir L, Halldorsson TI, Siggeirsdottir K, Cotch MF, Einarsdottir BO, Eiriksdottir G, Sigurdsson S, Launer LJ, Harris TB, Gudnason V, Sigurdsson G. PLoS One. 2014 Mar 12;9(3):e91122)

(Straube et al, 2009) (Straube S, Andrew Moore R, McQuay HJ. Vitamin D and chronic pain. *Pain* 2009; 141: 10–3)

(Sun et al, 2012) (Sun Q, Pan A, Hu FB, Manson JE, Rexrode KM. 25-Hydroxyvitamin D levels and the risk of stroke: a prospective study and meta-analysis. Stroke. 2012;43:1470–7)

(Urashima et al, 2010) (Urashima M, Segawa T, Okazaki M, Kurihara M, Wada Y, Ida H. Randomized trial of vitamin D supplementation to prevent seasonal influenza A in schoolchildren. Am J Clin Nutr. 2010;91:1255–60)

(Vit D, blueberries, 2013) (Synergistic induction of human cathelicidin antimicrobial peptide gene expression by vitamin D and stilbenoids. Molecular Nutrition & Food ResearchArticle first published online: 14 SEP 2013 DOI: 10.1002/mnfr.201300266. Oregon State University)

(Vitamin D, Umbrella review, 2014) (Vitamin D and multiple health outcomes: umbrella review of systematic reviews and meta-analyses of observational studies and randomized trials. BMJ 2014;348:g2035)

(Vrieling et al, 2012) (Vrieling A, Hein R, Abbas S, Schneeweiss A, Flesch-Janys D, Chang-Claude J. Serum 25-hydroxyvitamin D and postmenopausal breast cancer survival: a prospective patient cohort study. Breast Cancer Res. 2011;13(4):R74)

(Wang et al, 2008) (Wang TJ, Pencina MJ, Booth SL, et al. Vitamin D deficiency and risk of cardiovascular disease. *Circulation* 2008; 117: 503–11)

(Wiseman, 1993) (Wiseman H. Vitamin D is a membrane antioxidant. Ability to inhibit iron-dependent lipid peroxidation in liposomes compared to cholesterol, ergosterol and tamoxifen and relevance to anticancer action. FEBS Lett. 1993 Jul 12;326(1-3):285-8)

(Witham et al, 2009) (Witham MD, Nadir MA, Struthers AD. Effect of vitamin D on blood pressure: a systematic review and meta-analysis. J Hypertens. 2009;27:1948–54)

(Wolf et al, 2007) (Wolf M, Shah A, Gutierrez O, et al. Vitamin D levels and early mortality among incident hemodialysis patients. *Kidney Int* 2007; 72: 1004–13)

(Working group, 2005) (Working Group of the Australian and New Zealand Bone and Mineral Society, Endocrine Society of Australia, Osteoporosis Australia. Vitamin D and adult bone health in Australia and New Zealand: a position statement. *Med J Aust* 2005; 182: 281–5)

(Youssef et al, 2011) (Youssef DA, Miller CW, El-Abbassi AM, Cutchins DC, Cutchins C, Grant WB, Peiris AN. Antimicrobial implications of vitamin D. Dermatoendocrinol. 2011;3:220–9)

(Zipitis et al, 2008) (Zipitis CS, Akobeng AK. Vitamin D supplementation in early childhood and risk of type 1 diabetes: a systematic review and meta-analysis. Arch Dis Child. 2008;93:512–7)

Companion Books of Prof. R. Howes, MD, PhD:

Howes, R. M. *U.T.O.P.I.A. - Unified Theory of Oxygen Participation in Aerobiosis.* © 2004. Free Radical Publishing Co. Kentwood, LA, available at www.iwillfindthecure.org.

Howes R. M. *The Medical and Scientific Significance of Oxygen Free Radical Metabolism.* © 2005. Free Radical Publishing Co. Kentwood, LA. USA. available at www.iwillfindthecure.org.

Howes, R. M. *Hydrogen Peroxide Monograph 1: Scientific, Medical and Biochemical Overview.* © 2006; Free Radical Publishing Co. USA. 200 pages. available at www.iwillfindthecure.org.

Howes, R. M. Monograph 2: *Antioxidant vitamins A, C & E: Equivocal Scientific Studies,* © 2006; Free Radical Publishing Co. USA. 171 pages. available at www.iwillfindthecure.org.

Howes, R. M. *Cardiovascular Disease and Oxygen Free Radical Mythology,* © 2006;

Free Radical Publishing Co. USA. 308 pages. available at www.iwillfindthecure.org.

Howes, R. M. *Diabetes and Oxygen Free Radical Sophistry,* © 2006;

Free Radical Publishing Co. USA. Free Radical Publishing Co. USA. 366 pages. available at www.iwillfindthecure.org.

Howes, R. M. *Reactive Oxygen Species Insufficiency (ROSI)*

as the Basis for Disease Allowance and Coexistence:

Extraordinary Support for an Extraordinary Theory

Vol I, II & III. © 2008; 1564 pages. available at www.iwillfindthecure.org.

Howes, R. M. Volume I 501 pages #7 © 2008. Free Radical Publishing Co. USA.

Howes, R. M. Volume II 505 pages #8 © 2008. Free Radical Publishing Co. USA.

Howes, R. M. Volume III 562 pages #9 © 2008. Free Radical Publishing Co. USA.

Howes, R. M. *THE HOWES PAPERS*

© 2009; Free Radical Publishing Co. USA. 211 pages

Howes R.M. *"COFFEE TABLE MUSINGS of the*

Da Vinci in COWBOY BOOTS"

Pithy Prose and Perspicacious Aphorisms. © 2009; 103 pages

Howes, R. M. Reactive Oxygen Species vs. Antioxidants:

"The Oxypocalypse" or

"The war that never was" © 2010; Free Radical Publishing Co. USA. 550 pages. available at www.iwillfindthecure.org.

Howes R.M. *Death in Small Doses?:*

Antioxidant Vitamins A, C & E in the 21st Century

Book One: *A Health Impact Statement For The Layman*

© 2010; Trafford Publishing. Indianapolis, USA. 90 pages

Howes R.M. *Antioxidant Vitamins are Making A Killing;*

Antioxidant Vitamins A, C & E in the 21st Century

Book Two: *A Health Impact Statement For The Medical Scientist*

© 2010; 184 pages

- **Death In Small Doses? Trafford Publishing, © 2010**

- **Antioxidant Overkill, CreateSpace and Free Radical Publishing, © 2011**

- **Dangers of Excessive Antioxidants in Cancer Patients, CreateSpace and Free Radical Publishing, © 2011**

- Heart Disease and Antioxidant Failures, CreateSpace and Free Radical Publishing, © 2011

- Antioxidant Failures and Dangers, CreateSpace and Free Radical Publishing, © 2011

- Anti-Aging Anti-oxidant Scams, CreateSpace and Free Radical Publishing, © 2011

- Sports, Athletes, Exercise Facts and Antioxidant Myths, CreateSpace and Free Radical Publishing, © 2011

- Alzheimer's Disease: Forget Antioxidants and Supplements, CreateSpace and Free Radical Publishing, © 2012

- Sex, Performance, Reproduction, Naked Radicals And Antioxidants, CreateSpace and Free Radical Publishing, © 2012

- Antioxidants Linked To Deadly Unintended Consequences, CreateSpace and Free Radical Publishing, © 2013

- U.T.O.P.I.A.: Unified Theory of Oxygen Participation In Aerobiosis, CreateSpace and Free Radical Publishing, © 2014, revised

- Hydrogen Peroxide: A Health, Homeostatic and Protective Essentiality, CreateSpace and Free Radical Publishing, © 2014

- Reactive Oxygen Species vs. Antioxidants: The Oxypocalypse or The War That Never Was, CreateSpace and Free Radical Publishing, © 2014

- Diabetes and Oxygen Free Radical Sophistry, CreateSpace and Free Radical Publishing, © 2014, revised

- FISH OIL (Omega3 fatty acids): Facts, Fantasies & Failures. CreateSpace and Free Radical Publishing, © 2014

All books available at www.amazon.com; www.barnesandnobles.com; www.booksamillion.com.

Companion Papers of Prof. R. Howes, MD, PhD:

Dr. Howes has authored over 350 medical publications in health related editorials.

Citation: R. Howes: Mythology of Antioxidant Vitamins?. *The Journal of Evidence-Based Alternative and Complimentary Medicine.* April, 2011. 16(2): 149-189.

Citation: R. Howes: Cancer Therapy: A Review with Scientific Validation for the Role of Electronically Modified Oxygen Derivatives in Oncologic Treatment Modalities. *The Internet Journal of Alternative Medicine.* 2010 Volume 8 Number 1.

Citation: R. Howes: Hydrogen Peroxide: A review of a scientifically verifiable omnipresent ubiquitous essentiality of obligate, aerobic, carbon-based life forms. *The Internet Journal of Plastic Surgery.* 2010 Volume 7 Number 1.

Howes M.D., PhD., R. (2009). Dangers of Antioxidants in Cancer Patients: A Review. *PHILICA.COM Article number 153.* Published 7th February, 2009. (20 pages)

Howes M.D., PhD., R. (2008). Aging and anti-aging claims: a review on antioxidant vitamins A, C & E. *PHILICA.COM Article number 116.* Published on 12th January, 2008. (16 pages)

Howes M.D., PhD., R. (2007). Sleep: An original "radical" proposal. *PHILICA.COM Observation number 42.* Published on 5th October, 2007. (1 page)

Howes M.D., PhD., R. (2007). Antioxidant Vitamins A, C & E; Death in Small Doses and Legal Liability? *PHILICA.COM Article number 89.* Published on 5th April, 2007. (23 pages)

Howes M.D., PhD., R. (2007). Cancer, Apoptosis and Reactive Oxygen Species: A New Paradigm. *PHILICA.COM Article number 86.* Published on 26th February, 2007. (11 pages)

Howes M.D., PhD., R. (2007). Antioxidant Vitamins A, C and E: Assessing Potential for Harm. *PHILICA.COM Article number 83.* Published on 15th February, 2007. (14 pages)

Prof Randolph M. Howes MD,PhD

Howes M.D., PhD., R. (2007). The Consequent Downfall of the Free Radical Theory. *PHILICA.COM Article number 75*. Published on 22nd January, 2007. (9 pages)

Howes, R.M.: "The Free Radical Fantasy," The Annals of New York Academy of Sciences, 2006, Vol. 1067, pp. 22-26.

(Howes, 2005) (Howes, R.M. Tumoricidal Activity of An Injectable Singlet Oxygen System Generated From Physiological Agents: The Howes Singlet Oxygen Cancer Therapy System). In The Medical and Scientific Significance of Oxygen Free Radical Metabolism. © 2005. Free Radical Publishing Co. Kentwood, LA. pp. 893-912).

(Howes, Farber, 2005) (Howes, R.M. and Farber, G. Tumoricidal Activity of the Howes Singlet Oxygen Delivery System in Human Basal Cell Carcinoma. In The Medical and Scientific Significance of Oxygen Free Radical Metabolism. © 2005. Free Radical Publishing Co. Kentwood, LA. pp. 883-892).

(Howes et al, 1977) (Howes, R.M., Steele, R.H. and Hoopes, J.E., The role of Electronic excitation states in collagen biosynthesis, Persp. In Biol. And Med., Summer 1977, 20; 4:539-544).

(Howes, Steele, 1976) (Howes, R.M., Steele, R.H. and Hoopes, J.E., Peroxide induced Chemiluminescence in an in vitro proline hydroxylation system, 1976, 8; 1:77-84).

(Howes et al, 1976) (Howes, R. M., Allen, R.C., Su, C.T. and Hoopes, J.E., Altered polymorphonuclear leukocyte bioenergetics in patients with thermal injury, the Surgical Forum, 1976, 27:558-560).

(Howes, Steele, 1972) (Howes, R.M. and Steele, R.H., Microsomal chemiluminescence induced by NADPH and its relation to aryl-hydroxylations, Res Commun. Chem. Path. Pharmacol., March 1972, 3; 2:349-357).

(Howes, Steele, 1971) (Howes, R. M. and Steele, R. H., Microsomal chemiluminescence induced by NADPH and its relation to lipid peroxidation, Res. Commun. Chem. Path. Pharmacol., July-Sept. 1971, 2; 4 & 5:619-626).

I despise precious time wasted,
for it alone, is the unfinished canvas
displaying the portrait of my life.
R. M. Howes, M.D., Ph.D.
9/7/09

"We are what we repeatedly do. Excellence then, is not an act, but a habit." ~Aristotle

OTHER BOOKS

PUBLISHED: Partial list. The Fire Eaters, Molding your own destiny more easily, Carnivore Press, © 1982

Uplift, The Answer Book to your plastic and cosmetic surgery questions, Carnivore Press, © 1986

The Pundit Speaks, vol. I. An Anthology of Neoclassical Poetic Philosophy, Carnivore Press, © 1990

The Pundit Speaks, Volume II, An Anthology of Neoclassical Poetic Philosophy, Free Radical Press, © 1994

The Pundit Speaks, Volume III, An Anthology of Neoclassical Poetic Philosophy, Free Radical Press, © 1996

The Pundit Speaks, Volume IV, An Anthology of Neoclassical Poetic Philosophy, Free Radical Press, © 2000

The Fable of the Chocolate Covered Strawberry Coloring Book, Free Radical Press, © 2001

The Pundit Speaks, Volume IV, An Anthology of Neoclassical Poetic Philosophy, Free Radical Press, © 2003

The Pundit Speaks, Volume V, An Anthology of Neoclassical Poetic Philosophy, Trafford Publishing, © 2009

Coffee Table Musings of The DaVinci In Cowboy Boots, Trafford Publishing,© 2010

Available at: www.philica.com
www.medi.philica.com
www.iwillfindthecure.org
www.amazon.com

If you believe the implausible,
you will accept the indefensible and
not recognize the inexcusable.
R. M. Howes, M.D., Ph.D.
6/5/11

DOC
R ^{ANDOLPH}
HOWES

RAD!CAL

"Future's shape is sculpted by the persistent kneading hands of the impossible dreamer."
R. M. Howes, M.D., Ph.D.
5/2/04